TUNE YOUR BRAIN™

D1021385

Most Berkley Books are available at special quantity discounts for bulk purchases for sales promotions, premiums, fund-raising or educational use. Special books, or books excerpts, can also be created to fit specific needs.

For details, write to Special Markets, The Berkley Publishing Group, 200 Madison Avenue, New York, New York 10016.

TUNE YOUR BRAIN™

Using Music to Manage Your
Mind, Body, and Mood

Elizabeth Miles

Pacific
WITHDRAWN
University

Berkley Books / New York

PACIFIC UNIVERSITY
LIBRARY

This book is an original publication of The Berkley Publishing Group.

TUNE YOUR BRAIN

A Berkley Book / published by arrangement with the author

PRINTING HISTORY
Berkley trade paperback edition / October 1997

All rights reserved.
Copyright © 1997 and ™ by Elizabeth Miles.
Text design by Richard Oriolo.
This book may not be reproduced in whole or in part,
by mimeograph or any other means, without permission.
For information address: The Berkley Publishing Group, a member of Penguin Putnam Inc.,
200 Madison Avenue, New York, New York 10016.

The Putnam Berkley World Wide Web site address is http://www.berkley.com

ISBN: 0-425-16017-3

BERKLEY®
Berkley Books are published by The Berkley Publishing Group, a member of Penguin Putnam Inc.,
200 Madison Avenue, New York, New York 10016.
BERKLEY and the "B" design
are trademarks belonging to Berkley Publishing Corporation.

PRINTED IN THE UNITED STATES OF AMERICA
10 9 8 7 6 5 4 3 2 1

To my parents,
who attended all my concerts
despite the sometimes deleterious braintuning effects
and remained calm when my clarinet made the dog howl

Acknowledgments

··

I'm grateful to all the music teachers and band members who have been tuning my brain for years. From Miss Grady, my first-grade piano teacher, to my mentors and colleagues at the Department of Ethnomusicology at UCLA, thank you for all your accumulated knowledge of how music works and why it matters.

This book wouldn't exist without the research conducted by scholars in neurology, psychology, medicine, music therapy and ethnomusicology. May your fine work continue with renewed public interest and support.

The musical passion of many people in the record industry has helped inspire me to bring this idea to fruition. Thanks to Albert Imperato for his early and ongoing support; to Glenn Petry for his wise and invaluable discographical suggestions; to Kiku Loomis for savvy advice of many kinds; and to all the record companies that have helped make the discographies current and accurate, and whose ongoing efforts to record a wide variety of wonderful music make *Tune Your Brain* possible.

I have relied utterly on the love, support, and literary chops of my volunteer editorial team: Lindsay Clare, Liatris Cottam, Sarah Hendon, Bob Kramer, Tamara Loomis, James McGuire, Deenya Rabius, and Sarah Schiller. I also feel blessed by the enthusiastic and nationwide response to my braintuning survey; thanks to all who shared their personal experiences with me. Many others have offered ideas and encouragement that kept the spark burning every day.

My agent, Laurens Schwartz, believed in this project first; thank you for your faith. My editor, Barry Neville, made this project real. For your creative energy, thoughtful élan, and expressive skills, thanks especially to you.

Contents

....

Braintuning Basics: Music in Your Mind and Body

Have you ever put on music to get psyched up for an important presentation or exam, relax after a hectic day, exercise, set a romantic mood, think through a difficult problem, or celebrate a personal victory? Chances are, the answer is yes. Chances are that you are a music user.

There's nothing wrong with that—no shame, harm to your health, or fear of addiction. Using music is as natural as breathing or sleeping, and while many people do so instinctually, recent research indicates that the systematic use of music can be an effective way to consciously manage your mind, body, and mood.

From the discovery that listening to Mozart can raise your IQ to clinical trials showing that music can improve your memory, regulate vital signs like your heart rate and blood pressure, control your pain, change your emotional outlook, and direct your mental and physical energy levels throughout the day, science is finding that music can be a tool for better performance and health.

Tune Your Brain was born because the evidence supporting music as a method for self-enhancement exists, but nobody had collected and applied it to daily life. Until now, our knowledge of music's impact on the mind and body was splintered into different academic disciplines whose exclusivity prevented drawing practical conclusions. This book seeks to bridge that gap by synthesizing recent findings in neurology, psychology, medicine, and music therapy with an ethnomusicological understanding of music's time-honored applications in indigenous cultures around the world.

The result is the first guide to using the music *you like best* to motivate your mind and body for whatever you need to do. Wake up. Go to sleep. Brainstorm. Concentrate. Remember. Convince someone of something or assimilate new information. Socialize. Exercise. Beat stress. Heal. Control overeating and substance abuse. With the techniques available in this book, your favorite music can help you solve your problems, protect your health, and optimize your performance in all areas of life.

Music Uses You

Music wallpapers our consciousness in twentieth-century America. It permeates the background in offices, stores, restaurants, films, health clubs, waiting rooms, and airplanes. Like fast food, we tend to allow prefabricated music programming to determine our musical diet.

Just as fast food can be less nourishing than a fresh and natural menu, the music served to you in your daily life might have imbalances and deficiencies that detract from your maximum potential. Any time you listen to music that someone else has chosen, you are allowing other people to color your mood and control your body and mind.

You'll become a more proficient music user as you learn how music has helped people do everything from fight cancer pain to wait more patiently in line at the bank. You'll explore the mood difference between Mozart and Mahler . . . Nirvana and the Beatles . . . Brazilian *bateria* and Balinese *gamelan*. Discographies and music-mood quizzes in every chapter make it easy to match your personal preferences with the state you wish to attain, and because the system draws upon the whole world of music, you can choose from the sounds and styles you like the most. From doing higher math to having better sex, *Tune Your Brain* helps you transform your CD collection into a resource for personal well-being.

The following chapters explain what to listen to and how in order to:

- **Energize:** Wake up, prepare for performance and confrontations, recharge, exercise, get cheap and legal thrills

- **Relax:** Manage stress and anxiety, go to sleep, gain patience and people skills, control panic attacks, meditate, eat more slowly, speak more freely

- **Focus:** Enhance your IQ, facilitate memory and learning, concentrate, and prolong your attention span

- **Heal:** Overcome pain, recover from illness or injury, stimulate your immune system, stay calm during medical procedures and surgery

- **Uplift:** Break bad moods, treat depression, escape from negative thought patterns, fight chronic overeating, overcome shyness

- **Cleanse:** Vent feelings and frustrations to manage aggression and repressed anger, face grief, and handle problem relationships

- **Create:** Solve problems, access right-brain imagery, adopt creative habits for more innovative work and play, enrich your sex life

In addition to scientific research, *Tune Your Brain* draws on a nationwide survey of people from all walks of life that asked them how they use music. Throughout the book you'll read case studies and examples of these people applying braintuning techniques in their lives. Some are direct quotes; others are composites created to illustrate concepts in action. Many respondents shared the feeling that music was a very important part of their lives, but they weren't always exactly sure how or why. It's the goal of this book to help you discover the scientific and emotional underpinnings of your relationship with music and put them to work in making your daily life better.

Music in Your Mind

Hearing from Your Inner Ear

Music's impact on your mind and body begins with the physiological process of hearing. The ear is the first sensory organ to develop in the womb, preceding even the nervous system—so sound is your first source of information about the world. Once you're born, the primary function of the auditory system is orientation and self-defense. Your entire hearing apparatus is designed to detect, locate, and identify sound, then integrate these signals into propulsive behavior for self-preservation—for instance, fleeing from the woolly mammoth you hear charging from the rear. From an evolutionary standpoint, hearing is life itself, and as such, we were given a sophisticated system for processing sound in the brain, body, and nervous system.

Here's how hearing works: Sound waves in the air are captured by your outer ear—the part you can clean with a Q-Tip—and funneled into your middle ear. There, they vibrate tiny bones called ossicles, high-tech audio hardware that amplifies the sound two times over and passes it on to the inner ear. This is where things start to get interesting.

The *cochlea* of the inner ear is a fluid-filled coil lined with neurons in the form of tiny hair cells, each of which is tuned to a different frequency. The sound waves find the neurons matching their own frequency and make them vibrate. The cochlea then converts the *mechanical* energy of the ear-drum's vibration into *electrical* energy and transmits it into the brain. This means that every sound you hear sends actual electrical impulses directly into your mind. In other words, your inner ear transforms sound waves in the air into electricity in your body.

Once inside your brain, these electrical impulses move through the brain stem, the oldest layer of the brain and the locus of your instinctual responses, such as getting out of that mammoth's way before your conscious awareness of the sound of its charge has even kicked in. Here, musical energy activates the *limbic system*, structures such as the hypothalamus, hippocampus, amygdala, and parts of the thalamus that wrap around the brain stem and control your emotions. Music's effect on the limbic system is part of why certain pieces can make you happy or sad, and it also may explain the relationship medical researchers have found between music listening and hormonal balance. Finally, after generating motor responses, emotions, and hormones, music moves upward into the conscious part of your brain, the *auditory cortex*.

Like the cochlea, the auditory cortex contains cells corresponding to different sound frequencies, which are all mapped out on neural tissue. The electrical impulses activate these neurons, which encode the signals as recognizable sound.[1]

The development of brain-mapping technology has enabled recent breakthroughs in tracing music's pathways through the mind. Most importantly, researchers have identified elaborate neural networks in the cortex, called *feature detectors*, that process music. Some such networks might be tuned to musical intervals such as octaves, fourths, and fifths; others might specialize in detecting ascending and descending patterns. There may even be entire circuits linked together to encode familiar melodies. Furthermore, these networks are probably not hardwired, but programmable, or changeable by how much and what types of music you listen to. This would mean that the music you listen to actually determines the arrangement of neural networks in your brain.[2]

Brain-Mapping in Action

Neuroscientists are now using magnetic resonance imaging (MRI), positron emission tomography (PET), and electroencephalographs (EEG) to see which parts of the brain light up (receive blood or register increased electrical activity) during remembering, learning, thinking, listening to music, and other cognitive functions. These technologies have finally allowed brain research to be conducted on live human subjects—a boon to understanding the mental impact of music. Rats may run a mean maze, but they'll never appreciate a good jazz band.

EEG studies show that listening to music increases coherence, or electrical relationships, between different areas of the brain.[3] Evidence of electro-musical networks is also seen by activating different brain cell groups with an electrode, which can actually cause people to *hear* different fragments of song.[4]

Computer modeling also supports the existence of music maps in the mind. Physicist Gordon Shaw built a computer model of how cells in the auditory cortex might fire during learning. He translated the resulting mathematical code into sounds, and guess what? The model generated musical themes.[5] Could cell connections in the auditory cortex compose the brain's basic neural language?

Also known as neural modules or auditory-cognitive neural architecture, these neural networks perform a variety of sophisticated tasks that include encoding and remembering melodies, recognizing patterns, and filling in any missing musical elements like the fundamental or home tone of a series or chord, or a note's higher or lower octave equivalent.[6]

As neural networks accomplish these jobs, mostly through interactions between the frontal and temporal areas of the brain, they start trying to predict musical events based on what they've already processed and relate what's happening now to the music a few bars back. It's something like using the RAM on a computer, and is the same process of detecting and predicting patterns that underlies many cognitive processes. As brain cells fire across the synapses between them, they bridge the gap and make the connection easier the next time. Neuroscientists propose that as you listen to music, these connections form patterns that build themselves up to process information more efficiently, and so boost your cognitive powers.

Some of these networks seem to be solely dedicated to music, while others are shared with language, spatial-temporal reasoning, and movement. This circuit-sharing implies that music can enhance your abilities in these other areas—and also might influence other mental processes that we don't yet understand. By activating the right networks, listening to your favorite tunes could help you work with words, do math, and make a better play on the football field.

These new discoveries about music come at a time when neuroscientists are rethinking the nature of intelligence. Scholars like Gerald Edelman and William Calvin propose that intelligence develops when stimulation (like music) strengthens certain neural circuits and pathways, developing a kind of softwired syntax of the mind that enables high-level communication and abstract thought.[7] MIT composer David Epstein bases a theory on Edelman's work proposing that music, as a continually varied succession of patterns, represents how the brain learns to think.[8] Music researcher W. Jay Dowling theorizes that the pattern recognition involved in listening to music engages "procedural" memory and so adds to the store of motor and perceptual skills that constitute "implicit" knowledge.[9] In general, neuroscience is leaning toward the notion that the ongoing creation of neural circuitry shapes our very consciousness.

Left Brain–Right Brain

The discovery of music's neural impact is exciting, but music might derive even more cognitive power from its unique ability to access both the left and right hemispheres of the brain. Maybe you think of yourself as left brain if you're an analytical or word-driven type, or right brain if you're creative or visual. In general, the left brain handles symbolic activities, like language and logic, while the right brain is responsible for direct perception, including spatial tasks and abstract, intuitive leaps. Listening to music actually taps both sides, potentially uniting creative and analytical functions in the mind.

The Corpus Callosum: Your Interhemispheric Information Superhighway

The two sides of your brain are physically separated, like halves of a walnut. The only reason that your right hand knows what your left hand is doing is the *corpus callosum*, a bundle of fifty million nerve fibers joining one hemisphere to the other, somewhat like the coaxial cable that links your computer to the Internet.

Studies of adults who received early musical training show that their corpus callosums are larger than average, indicating increased interhemispheric traffic as a result of all that music processing.[10] Evidence suggests that music can actually increase communication between both sides of the brain, allowing you to join logic and insight in all your cognitive endeavors. Let music increase the speed limit on your own information superhighway.

Music and language circuits are found in both cerebral hemispheres, mostly in temporal lobes that do the lower-order work of music and speech cognition. For higher-order workings, past research has postulated that music is mostly processed in the right side of the brain, while the left takes care of language—a theory supported by studies of patients with damaged left brains who can't speak but can still make or perceive music, and, on the flip side, those with damaged right brains who are amusical but still able to speak. And indeed, neurologists agree that the left side of the brain has regions dedicated to language, while areas of the right side specialize in music.[11]

But the theory of right-brain dominance for musical functions might be up for grabs. A team of German neurologists think they've found the center for perfect pitch on the left side,[12] and we now know that recognition and analysis of melody, rhythm, and intervals are left-brain activities. Despite the existence of specialized areas for language on the left and music on the right, many scientists are beginning to explore music processing as a bilateral activity that operates on both sides of the brain[13]—maybe even as a higher function than language. Perhaps a more advanced way of knowing, analyzing, synthesizing, and communicating than we currently find in speech, music might offer the power to harmonize the cerebral hemispheres.

Music might offer the power to harmonize the cerebral hemispheres.

Listening from Both Sides of the Brain

When you listen to music, the right brain essentially receives the big picture and the left brain analyzes the details. The functions of both hemispheres are necessary to your comprehension and enjoyment of music.[14]

Left Brain

- Analyzing and recognizing sequences and form

- Interval judgments (harmonies)

- Identifying familiar tunes

- Perfect pitch

- Recognizing and repeating rhythms (temporal sequencing)

- Dynamics (changes in volume)

Right Brain

- Implicit cognition or perceiving the "big picture"

- Pitch judgments

- Processing new melodic sequences and implied harmonic relations

- Perceiving overtones to distinguish between timbres

- Imagining or mentally generating music

Left and Right Brain

◊ ◊ ◊ ◊ ◊ Singing familiar tunes ◊ ◊ ◊ ◊ ◊

Now throw this into the mix: The degree to which you lateralize music processing, or push it to one side of the brain or the other, might vary with time of day, gender, and simply from one person to the next—and the whole thing could be reversed if you're left-handed.[15]

It should be noted that though several braintuning techniques in this book incorporate the idea of hemisphere specialization, cognitive processes are complex and may draw on many parts of the brain. The references to left- and right-brain activities are general and meant to describe usual patterns of cerebral specialization rather than exclusive localization.

No matter the hemisphere, music can shape your neural topography for the better, and you don't need to be a neuroscientist to put it to work for you.

Quantum Music?

Neurologists aren't the only scientists currently placing music under the microscope; some new theories are also coming from the field of physics. Nobel laureate physicist Brian Josephson views music like atoms in terms of quantum theory, proposing parallels between DNA and musical ideas, and theorizing that music activates a primary level of consciousness.

Music's quantum power, argues Josephson, lies in its ability to "pump the system"—exposing atoms to musical electricity, which makes them able to emit more energy than they absorb. He further likens the balance-imbalance condition in biosystems to the tension and release patterns found in music, suggesting that music models the maintenance of balance for the human organism.[16]

Music theorist Roger Hyde proposes an evolutionary theory—that music might be our most recently evolved capacity, residing in our very freshest layer of brain. By helping us to detect and predict patterns, it might even function as our latest software upgrade, transcending the verbal and visual structures in the brain that have brought us through these early evolutionary stages.[17]

Sound Waves Make Brain Waves

In addition to rearranging your neural networks, music plays with your state of mind as the electrical energy generated by firing neurons creates *brain waves*. The alpha, beta, theta, and delta frequencies created by neural activity—brain waves—determine what operations you're best suited to conduct at the moment. For instance, alpha states, which correlate with relaxation, make the brain receptive to new information, focus your mind for quiet thought, and enable meditation. Beta is best for attentive mental activity. Theta waves indicate stress, pleasure deprivation, or creative effort. Slow the waves to delta speed and you're asleep. The music you listen to can influence the waves' frequency, and so your state of mind.

Once it's done with your mind, music sets to work on the state of your body. Musical messages travel down your spinal cord, impacting the *auto-*

nomic nervous system that regulates your heart rate, blood pressure, muscular activity, metabolism, and other vital functions. Your autonomic nervous system is literally the link between your mental and physical self, and music directly affects its workings.

Brain Waves

Brain waves measure the electrical activity in your brain, which determines the kind of mental work you can do best—and which can be altered with music.[18] Here are the approximate speeds of brain waves in cycles per second (cps):

- **Beta (13–30 cps)** Attentive mental activity; coping with external stimuli; quick response, immediate problems, and juggling many thoughts at once.

- **Alpha (8–13 cps)** Quiet, focused concentration.

- **Theta (4–9 cps)** Creativity and imagery, as well as stress, frustration, and disappointment.

- **Delta (less than 6 cps)** Deep sleep.

Music in Your Body

Music As Autonomic Weapon

The autonomic nervous system regulates your vital signs, indicators such as heart rate, pulse, blood pressure, breathing, and the electrical activity of muscles that measure your arousal level and determine your physical readiness for various activities. The first published American experiment with music's effect on the autonomic nervous system was a 1924 study of the electrocardiograms (EKGs) and blood pressure of people listening to music.[19] Since then, decades of research in music therapy have linked listening to music with autonomic nervous system responses, as well as internal secretions and activity in the sympathetic nervous system (a subdivision of the autonomic system).

In general, fast, rhythmic, loud music leads to physiological arousal—increases in the measures of autonomic nervous system activity—and slow, soft music encourages relaxation, or decreases in these measures. Experimenters have been able to drive people's pulse rates by manipulating the music's volume and speed. It's also been found that your breathing tends to synch up, or entrain, to the music's beat at a ratio that works for your body, and will then change with the music's tempo. People entrain at different ratios, and you could be more likely to synchronize either your pulse or your breathing, depending upon whether you're a circulatory reactor (pulse) or a respiratory reactor (breathing).

Music also affects the electrical activity, or action potential, in your muscles. Hand grip squeeze tests have found that your grip weakens to lullabies and strengthens to marches. Different types of music seem to send action potentials into different muscles in the body.

Autonomic Audio

Music can be used to direct autonomic functions including:

- Heart rate

- Pulse

- Breathing (speed, depth, and rhythm)

- Blood pressure (diastolic and systolic)

- Muscle tension and action potential

- Galvanic skin response[20]

Although the general rule is that loud, fast music speeds you up and soft, slow music puts on the brakes, your personal response to music also depends upon your autonomic reactivity, determined by things like your age, gender, and physical fitness, as well as your emotional reactivity and personal attitude toward the music. So the degree of autonomic response to any given piece of music can vary from one person to the next.

Experiments gauging the cognitive and behavioral changes associated with music listening have found that stimulating music and physiological arousal are associated with increased energy, aggression, and anxiety, while soothing music and relaxation can lead to calmness, passivity, and depression.

You don't have to actually hear to be affected by music at the autonomic level. Even deaf mutes show physiological responses to the vibrations of musical sound. Evidence indicates that even in the absence of the *sense* of hearing to process sound, the human body has an innate *sensibility* to music that reaches to the deepest core.

Got Rhythm? Your Circadian Hormonal Cycles

Rhythm—you have it when you breathe, speak, walk, or run. You have it when your heart beats and your blood pulses in your arteries. Rhythm is the regulating meter of human life.

The solar system has rhythm, too—the regular rising and setting of the sun that times our days on earth. You're probably well aware that your mind and body follow natural energy cycles that get you out of bed and off to work feeling fresh and alert in the morning, then draw you, drained and tired, back to rest at night. What you might not know is that these cycles corresponding to light and dark, wakefulness and sleep, are governed by a complex system of hormones released in your body throughout the day. Secretions of corticotrophin-releasing hormone (CRH), adrenocorticotrophic hormone (ACTH), and cortisol wake you up in the morning; melatonin puts you to sleep at night. A substance called NPY makes you crave carbohydrates at breakfast time, while galanin stimulates your desire for fatty foods for dinner. Your hormone balance, body temperature, electrolytes, and brain chemistry all change with the clock in a preprogrammed chronobiological sequence. Called *circadian rhythms*, your daily energy cycles are natural, but they don't always synchronize with your schedule.

You might know some of your own biorhythmic idiosyncrasies: perhaps a midmorning energy rush, afternoon slump, or spurt of late-night juice. If everyone had parallel circadian rhythms, we would all feel the same at various times of day, allowing us to share our swings with everybody else. But it isn't so simple. Your unique temperament and biology interact with your daily schedule of secretions to make your circadian self all your own. You are alone in your energies.

The right music can affect your hormonal secretions and, working in tandem with autonomic functions, can help realign your biorhythms with your energy needs.[21] People have long used music to suit their state of mind to their schedules. From the Indian *raga* system, in which the sound of the scale changes from morning to night to create moods appropriate to the time of day, to ancient and contemporary repertoires all around the world that include work songs to wake up and motivate, dance music to recreate, and lullabies to go to sleep, music is universally used as a tool to regulate internal rhythms.

Here's an example of how you can use the techniques in the following chapters to manage your circadian cycles during a typical day:

When Your Circadian Rhythms Say:	The Braintuning Solution:
7 AM "YAWN." Your mind and body may be most alert first thing in the morning, but your sleepy nervous system often needs a jump start to catch up.	Use an **energizing** selection to prime your physiology and take wakeful advantage of your peak-performance morning hours.
10 AM "YOW!" You finish your staff meeting on a morning energy high—in fact, you're too agitated about the proposed restructuring to concentrate on the memo that could save your job.	Listen to a **focusing** selection through headphones to direct your thoughts to the task at hand, and screen out the juicy but distracting gossip over at the copy machine.
1 PM "BLAH." Your energy has peaked for the day, lunch is digesting in your stomach, and you're feeling blue and bored.	Take a walk around the block with an **uplifting** selection on your Walkman to raise your spirits and preempt an afternoon snooze.
3 PM "BLANK." You enter the classic mid-afternoon slump just when your boss asks for your input on a creative new fund-raising campaign.	Put on a **creating** selection to stimulate free association from the right hemisphere of your brain. Shower your boss with the results of your brainstorm.
6 PM "KILL!" You're stuck in traffic and late for your yoga class. Your stomach is churning after a stressful day, and you're in danger of harming a fellow motorist.	Blast a **cleansing** selection in your car stereo, scream along, and feel the adrenal hormones abate.
7 PM "GRR." You arrive home to find your husband laid out on the couch with a tension headache and a temper to match. You wonder why people mate for life.	Play some **healing** music to clear up his headache in time for a sensual dinner à deux.
11 PM "HELLO!" It's time for bed, but suddenly you're wide awake, worried about what you didn't do today and what tomorrow holds.	Cue up a **relaxing** selection on your bedside tape player, dim the lights, and let the musical massage lull you to sleep.

If your schedule demands steady, day-long performance, you probably already tried to control your circadian cycles with caffeine, alcohol, exercise, and mental effort. Music offers a natural way to keep your body in synch with your daily routines.

Music and Mood

Mood: Whatever Moves You

There's more to feeling your best than simply controlling your energy cycles. There are elusive emotional components, too: moods. Your emotional outlook is certainly impacted by your energy level—it's easy to feel happy when you're full of life or depressed when you're tired—but psychologists describe mood in broader terms that include:

- Physiological arousal levels (energy)

- Subjective, cognitive reactions (emotions)

- Behavioral responses (actions)

A variety of psychological scales have been developed to study mood, and they have shown music to be a powerful manipulator of your emotional state. Psychologists were using music to induce moods as early as 1806, when Samuel Mathews first proposed the iso principle, whereby you could induce mood by matching music to the patient's current mind-set—for instance, downbeat music for a depressed patient—then gradually changing the music's tempo, volume, pitch, melody, and rhythm until it approached the desired state.[22] Later developed to move people from sad to happy, restless to calm, bored to active, and active to majestic, the iso principle has become standard practice in mood induction,[23] and you'll see it utilized in several braintuning techniques.

Other studies have confirmed music's usefulness as a mood regulator. Kate Hevner's investigation of music's emotional effect led her to create a mood wheel, which designates the musical characteristics that cause people to feel spiritual, sad, dreamy, lyrical, playful, happy, excited, and vigorous. Another study found that inducing a good mood with music increased self-esteem, while yet another discovered that using music to bring on either elation or depression enhanced creativity. While several different kinds of experiments have supported music's mood-inducing effect, it has also been found that people tend to have the same emotional reactions to different kinds of music regardless of age or gender.[24]

Music, Mind, Body, and Mood

Music has a long history, through the ages and across cultures, as a treatment for mind, body, and mood. In the Western tradition, the history of music as a multifaceted "medicine" begins in ancient Egypt and continues through Pythagorus, Plato, and Aristotle into the present day. Indigenous cultures have accessed music's power since before written history began, and great civilizations from Confucian China to the Aztec empire developed sophisticated philosophies describing the music-mind-body connection. In the Middle East, each *maqam*, or scale, is thought to represent distinct ideological powers, expressive characters, and states of the soul. Similarly, Indian scale systems, or *ragas*, are considered to convey emotion and mood through their psychological or cosmological properties. In Irish folklore, music is conceptualized as the birth by a water goddess of three sons, Sorrow, Mirth, and Sleep—the states that music can induce. And the Chinese consider major keys to be *yang*—strong, masculine, and hard—and minor keys to be *yin*—soft, feminine, and weak. Finally, in Wisconsin, dairy farmers play music to cows to make them give more milk.

The Historical Hit Parade[25]

Prehistoric times   **The caveman** is the first documented musician. Singing was probably the first music prehistoric people made—it's difficult to pinpoint exactly when—and archaeologists have excavated bone flutes, bullroarers, rattles, and shakers dating back as far as the Paleolithic era.

Early history   **Indigenous cultures** all over the world, from Native Americans to Australian aborigines to African tribes, begin to develop repertoires of functional music for work, relaxation, healing, love, socializing, and spiritual ritual.

Ancient Egypt   The **Kahum papyrus** refers to healing the sick with song.

2697 B.C.   **Chinese legend** asserts that music begins when the emperor sends a man named Ling Lun to the western mountains to cut bamboo pipes that would sound the fundamental pitches required to harmonize the whole universe. Ling Lun's pipes need further fine-tuning by court musicians and astrologers in order to resonate with *all* the elements of nature and supernature.

Mythical times **Apollo**, leader of the Muses, is the god of music, medicine, and mental purity, so the Greek deities themselves bless the connection between mind, body, and music. Apollo's servant Orpheus plays a harp with magical healing powers with which he charms his way into Hades to rescue a goddess in distress.

C. 850 B.C. The Greek bard **Homer** recommends music to alleviate anger, sorrow, worry, fear, and fatigue, and claims that choral singing can prevent the plague. Other Greek physicians, philosophers, and historians recommending music as medicine include Thales of Miletus, Xenocrates, Theophratus, Diodorus Sicculus, Herophilus, Polybius, Aesclepiades of Bithynia, and Galen. The Greeks also use music to soothe mobs, vanquish enemies, calm violent tempers, cure hangovers, and heal various physical and mental illnesses.

580–500 B.C. The mathematician **Pythagorus**, the granddaddy of Western music theory, who discovered the physics of musical sound, advocates music as a daily requirement for good health. His followers come to him for rigorous mood-music treatments during which he uses tonality to manipulate their emotions and regulate their daily rhythms. (Rumor has it that Pythagorus might have learned his musical methods from the ancient Egyptians.)

551–479 B.C. **Confucius**, always a practical man, proclaims that music and ritual are necessary to harmonious living.

C. 428–348 B.C. The great philosopher **Plato** praises music's power to harmonize the revolutions of the soul when its rhythms have been disturbed. He advocates using music not for pleasure, but for the enhancement of perception and physical prowess: "All audible music sound is given us for the sake of harmony, which has motions akin to the orbits in our soul, and which, as anyone who makes intelligent use of the arts knows, is not to be used, as is commonly thought, to give irrational pleasure, but as a heaven-sent ally in reducing to order and harmony any disharmony in the revolutions within us."

Plato feels so strongly about music that he wants to ban specific modes that are sorrowful or encourage laziness or drinking.

384–322 B.C.   **Aristotle** concurs with his predecessors: Music provides an emotional catharsis with medicinal benefits.

106–43 B.C.   Roman statesman **Cicero** writes that "there is nothing so kindred to our feelings as rhythmic cadences and musical sounds, by which we are stimulated and inflamed and soothed and thrown into a state of languor, and often brought to a state of cheerfulness or sorrow."

Scriptural times   **David cures King Saul** of mental illness by playing his harp; **Elisha is healed** by a minstrel's song.

A.D. 1500s   **Indian artists** confirm the music-mood connection when they begin painting *ragamalas,* miniatures depicting thirty-six different *ragas* (musical scales), each with a different emotional setting.

The Renaissance   European thinkers begin the first documented discussion of **music's influence on breathing, blood pressure, muscular activity and digestion.**

A.D. 1730s   The Italian castrato Farinelli claims to **cure Spanish King Philip V of depression** by singing arias.

A.D. 1789   George Washington is elected president of the United States and an article entitled "Music Physically Considered," about **using music to treat depression** by exciting the nervous system, appears in the *Columbian* magazine. The author is the first American to propose in print that music's impact on the mind could treat the body and support overall health.

1800s   Americans and Europeans begin a course of **experimentation with the relationship between music and mental state** with the aim of discovering applications for psychiatric treatment. Physicians write that music presents a viable, "less life-threatening" alternative to traditional medicine. German philosopher Friedrich Nietzsche asks, "What is it that my whole body really expects of music? I believe, its own *ease*."

1804   American psychiatrist Edwin Atlee writes about **using music to treat mania** in "An Inaugural Essay on the Influence of Music in the Cure of Diseases."

1880–1903   Reports of **music's effect on cardiac output, respiratory rate, pulse, and blood pressure** roll in from Russia, France, and the United States.

1890s   Swiss educator **Emile Jaques-Dalcroze** formulates *eurhythmics*, a music and movement learning system that treats the body as a natural rhythmic instrument.

1899   **The first controlled music therapy experiment** is conducted by American neurologist James L. Corning, pertaining to sleep and the emotions.

Early 1900s   European composers and music educators **Carl Orff** and **Zoltán Kodály** discover a universal "Ur song" sung by children of all different cultures in their play. This sequence of the third, fifth, and sixth tones of the major scale seems to be given to humans by nature.

1914   American physician Evan O'Neill Kane reports **using music to alleviate pain in the hospital.**

1924   One of the first controlled American lab experiments quantifies music's effect on pulse rate, blood pressure, blood flow, and electrical activity in the heart—and **music is clinically validated as a medical treatment.**[26]

1940s   **Pioneering scientific studies** by psychologists and physicians in the United States discover that music can produce various moods, prolong attention span, relieve internal tension, stimulate associations and imagery, and facilitate self-expression.

The Music Research Foundation is founded to investigate the use of music in medical and psychiatric treatment. **Music therapy is born.**

1980s   Empirical studies of **music's clinical applications in medical settings** begin in earnest.

1993   Experimenters at the University of California at Irvine establish that **Mozart makes you smarter** with an experiment in which listening to Amadeus' piano sonata improved IQ by an average of nine points.

From the cave people to the neuroscientists of the 1990s, the consensus is clear: music can make a difference in how you feel, think, and act. But which music, why, and how?

In pre-Biblical times, thinkers such as Pythagorus and Plato understood that different kinds of music had different effects, but they couldn't have anticipated the dizzying array of musical styles available to us in the twentieth century. In fact, while music is one of the most ancient of human inventions, the ability to reproduce and listen to it at will is quite new. Thomas Edison invented his talking machine in 1877, which became the gramophone in 1897 and the electric phonograph in 1925. After millenia of making music, we've only been able to record and replay it for a century. Playback technology gives individuals unprecedented listening freedom but also bypasses the social conventions that used to ensure that the "right" music was presented for various occasions and needs. Now, your stereo system gives you the option of going into musical trance without attending a possession ceremony or rave, but this state of mind might not be your best bet if you're trying to finish up a financial analysis under deadline.

What Puts the Mood into Music?

The factors that determine a musical selection's psychophysiological effect include:

- Speed
- Volume
- Rhythm
- Instrumentation

- Timbre, or sound color (like an oboe versus a guitar)

- Texture, or how many parts there are and the way they're put together (a four-piece rock band versus a gospel chorus)

- Form

- Harmonic and melodic structure

- High or low pitch

For instance, as already mentioned, loud and fast music stimulates you, and slow and soft sounds are soothing. In addition, high pitches generally key you up and low ones relax you; syncopated or ragged rhythms are more stimulating than straight ones; symmetrical form and harmonic consonance require less attention than free or uneven forms or dissonance.

(See the glossary at the back of the book for further clarification of musical terms used throughout the text.)

The Heartbeat Effect

Though people make and enjoy music of all different speeds, there's a surprisingly coherent global consensus on what tempo seems comfortable or natural in music. Clinical trials, psychological studies, and surveys of music all over the world indicate that the most comfortable tempo is around eighty beats per minute—about the rate of the average human heartbeat.[27] Whether we're tuning into our inner rhythms or wishing for a return to the womb, people's feelings about musical speed seem to be quite organic.

Some of the braintuning techniques you'll see in coming chapters use the heartbeat effect, either taking advantage of the body's natural affinity for music at this tempo or recommending selections slower or faster than the heartbeat range to achieve various physiological and emotional goals. In the world of musical tempo, eighty beats per minute can be considered the golden mean.

The following chapters guide you through the process of choosing the right music to achieve the effect you want. The techniques are based on the impact that specific musical characteristics have been shown to have on your neural networks, brain waves, autonomic indicators, and so forth. But just as important to the braintuning concept and absent from much of the specially composed mood and meditation music on the market is *your personal preference*.

All the studies show that you are most deeply affected, in everything from your blood pressure to your hormonal secretions to your emotions and mood, by music *you like*.[28] So even if a recording is supposed to be scientifically designed to make you relaxed or alert or anything else (and beware the "science" of some of these products), if you don't like the sound, its effect will be small, and you're unlikely to incorporate the music into your daily life. Conversely, using your favorite recordings to optimize your health and performance is more effective, more efficient, and a lot more fun.

Braintuning Basics: Counting Beats per Minute

Some of the techniques in *Tune Your Brain* refer to beats per minute, a way of measuring tempo or speed in music. Though the discographies in each chapter are designed to guide you to music that moves at a speed appropriate to the mood state, you can count the beats per minute of any piece of music for use in specific braintuning applications:

- Put on the music and listen for the beat—the internal clock that ticks off the "seconds" of this particular selection. One easy way to find it is by tapping your foot. Each tap is a beat.

- Now, using the clock on your CD player or a watch with a second hand, count how many beats you hear in a minute. It can be hard to keep your concentration the first few times, as there tend to be many beats in a minute and the way we count (in tens) often doesn't correspond with the way beats are grouped (usually in fours). A little practice solves this problem. Your final count is the beats per minute, or bpm.

- There's a natural tendency to divide very slow beats in half or perceive fast ones in groups of two. This matters much less than how you perceive the beat—so count what you hear. If you can't find a beat at all, chances are the music is unmetered—a free form of rhythm encountered everywhere from Gregorian chant to avant-garde jazz. You won't come up with a bpm in such a case, but you can use your judgment to gauge the music's tempo and how it relates to your present braintuning application.

Personal Preference: From Grunge to Gamelan

Musical preference is a fairly complicated phenomenon, and research into its roots have identified many variables and feedback loops that form and re-form your tastes throughout your life. Before music even hits your ear it's filtered through the cultural conditioning of peers, family, authorities, and the media. Then it's processed by your individual auditory, cognitive, and emotional structures and interacts with personal characteristics like age, sex, ethnicity, personality, musical training, socioeconomic status, and your own store of memories. Once you decide you like something you might listen to it so much that you burn out and ultimately reject it—or it could become a lifelong favorite.

You don't have to be able to break music down into its components to like or dislike its individual elements. Even without the training to identify physical properties such as melody, harmony, rhythm, timbre, texture, or form, studies show that you can react as specifically as trained musicians to the properties that please or displease you. Some people will consistently prefer simple canons to five-part fugues, or vice versa, without even knowing what those two musical forms are. Musical preferences are strong—set, or at least separable, from parents' tastes by age ten—and can operate at a level more sophisticated than your own musical knowledge.[29]

Music preferences influence people even when they think they're behaving objectively. When a group of young adults were asked to scale the intensity of nine different samples of rock music, those who disliked the music perceived it as more intense than those who didn't. In a related study, subjects were given instructions for adjusting the volume of a music sample. Though everybody received the same instructions, those who liked the music turned it up higher than those who didn't.[30]

The world of music is as diverse as listeners' loyalties are strong. You can use your favorite music to enhance your daily life whether you prefer grunge rock or Balinese gamelan. Braintuning is about using your musical tastes to your own advantage.

The Braintuning Discographies

Each of the chapters in *Tune Your Brain* contains a discographical chart of recommended recordings organized by genre, so you can either go straight to the styles you like best or follow new musical paths to the desired state of mind. The design is meant to help you get more out of the music you love—and get you to know more music. There is also a Braintuning Five for each chapter, a quick list of five very diverse selections to get you started.

The discographies are intended to be both accessible and diverse, to make it as easy to find your favorites as it is to explore new directions. Because there are so many recordings available, the lists are inevitably a *very limited sampling*, usually with only one citation per artist and that often a "greatest hits" collection that serves well as an introduction to the musician, composer, or ensemble but might not please devoted fans. Use the listings as suggested starting places and explore from there, testing new selections with the music-mood quizzes to make sure they have the effect you want.

In world music, the discographies generally favor authentic native traditions over reinterpretations by Western musicians to allow you to tap directly into the music's original power. There are some exceptions, when adaptation either contributes to the music's mood effect or has created a new and distinct style that might contribute to your braintuning efforts.

Every attempt has been made to list only recordings that are widely available in CD format. Where appropriate, recordings that contain tracks representing more than one mood state have been cross-listed so that you can get the most braintuning benefits from each CD. There are now many ways to purchase CDs; refer to the Sources section on page 255 for more information.

The Music-Mood Tests

Everyone has a personal response to music governed by their autonomic reactivity, personal tastes, and past experience. Madonna might rev you up more than she does your mother—or vice versa.

The music-mood quizzes in each braintuning chapter enable you to "audition" individual recordings to determine their mood effect for you. Photocopy and use them on different selections and styles of music, then record your results in the accompanying journals to compile a personalized collection of braintuning tools.

The music-mood tests also enable you to explore beyond the recommended discographies. Maybe certain songs by Hole mellow you out; you won't find them mentioned in the Relax chapter, but there's no reason you shouldn't use them to fight stress if they pass the test.

The Music-Mood Tests: Instructions

Follow these instructions for all the music-mood tests in the book:

1. Choose a time when you feel you need the braintuning effect you're testing—for instance, first thing in the morning for an energizing selection, or during a stress attack for a relaxing piece.
2. Choose a selection to test and cue it up on your stereo system.
3. Rate your feelings before listening by assigning a score from 1 to 5 for each of the mood elements listed, using 1 for "not at all," 3 for "somewhat," and 5 for "very." Work quickly, choosing the first response that comes to mind.
4. Listen to your selection, following any relevant braintuning basics for listening in that mood state (for instance, use a comfortably loud level to energize and a moderate to soft volume to relax). If the piece is five minutes or less, listen to the whole selection; for longer pieces, listen to at least the first three to five minutes (try to stop at a natural breaking point).
5. Immediately rate your mood elements again.
6. Tabulate your change for each mood element and add them up. This is your mood response rating for this piece of music.
7. To interpret your score:

   31–40   Hot! This music is master of your mind, body, and mood.
   21–30   Very effective.
   11–20   Useful.
   0–10   Enjoy this music for itself, but not to affect your mood in this area.

Listening Modes

Most of the braintuning techniques distinguish between conscious and background listening. Music's effect on your mind and body tends to be more intense when you lend it your full attention, and this is often recommended. But when you're trying to focus on a task, manage ongoing stress, or facilitate social interaction, background listening is the way to go. The individual techniques will guide you.

For many Americans, conscious listening is a forgotten mode of music appreciation. We're so inured to background soundtracks that we rarely stop to pay full attention. If it seems strange when you first try focused listening, relax and remember that it requires no more attention than what you devote to conversation. You don't have to know the structure of a symphony to be a conscious listener any more than you need to know the recipe for a delicious dish to enjoy its taste.

Many braintuning techniques also call for a personal, portable CD or tape player with headphones. The ability to make your musical mood induction both mobile and private means you can integrate it into a wide variety of situations in your daily life. With a Walkman and headphones, for instance, you can be gearing up for a big sales call while your office mates destress.

Interestingly, musicians tend to have an even greater emotional and physiological response to music than nonexperts,[31] suggesting that becoming more aware of music might heighten its effect on you. In fact, studies have shown that melodic perception migrates from the right to the left brain as listeners become more adept and seek deeper analytical understanding of what they hear. Likewise, the braintuning techniques in this book may become even more powerful as you use them and thereby increase your musical awareness and develop the sophistication of your auditory cortex.

Music also has strong associative properties and a direct line to your memory, so over time, as you begin to associate "I Feel Good" with energizing for a presentation or "Art of the Fugue" with getting down to work, the mood effect of the music will be reinforced, and the recording will become an ever-better cue to induce the desired state. But if your presentation is a bust or the work session unproductive, you might attach the memory of failure to the music, which will then lose some or all of its potency in that braintuning application. Realizing that your brain is redesigning itself with every experience you have, retire or retest selections as necessary.

Why Tune Your Brain?

Even if you find the facts about music's impact on your life compelling, you might wonder, why bother? I've made it this far without consciously controlling my mood or my relationship with music. I might not be perfect, but I'm coping.

You know what happens when you don't tune up your car. The bill is inevitably high—as is the price of stress, fatigue, cloudy thinking, depression, unexpressed anger, alienation, boredom, inhibitions, and all the other limitations on your personal potential that you might write off to bad moods.

The long-term benefits of the mindful use of music in your life include:

- More energy

- Enhanced cognition

- Increased tolerance for stress and pressure

- Better health

- Ability to adapt to circumstances and rise to challenges

- Greater self-awareness, self-confidence, and feeling of personal control

- Alternatives to detrimental mind-altering habits

- Enhanced creativity

People make and listen to music for a wide variety of reasons that include its aesthetic, social, cultural, political, and historical meaning. This book takes an applied approach to music, which, by focusing on its measurable impact on your body and mind, begs many of these larger questions. They are extensively addressed elsewhere; so here, prepare to explore music's documented power to help you think, work, move, create, relax, and relate at your personal best.

One

Energize

Human energy is one of the most precious commodities on earth, and there's rarely enough to go around. The national coffee bar craze is proof that we live in an age of superachieving alertness, and those who snooze often suffer for it. Fortunately, a natural and nontoxic stimulus is close at hand. When you need peak performance, music can arouse your body, speed up your brain waves, and fill you with the electric energy of sound.

Energize Overview

Energizing Music Can Help You With:	Use These Techniques if You Are:	How Music Helps:
Waking Up	Tired, foggy, or short on sleep; a slow starter out of bed.	Stimulates your autonomic nervous system to speed up your vital signs.
Presentations and Performance	Preparing for a big sales pitch, meeting, speech, or stage appearance.	Gears up activity in muscles, nerves, and neural networks; clears your mind of fear.

Competition and Negotiations	Facing off—on the field, in the boardroom, in court.	Induces positive victory mood; stokes aggression; primes reflexes for quick decisions.
Recharge Breaks	Slowing down on the job, in the car, with the kids . . .	Restarts the muscular, nervous, and cardiac functions that slow down when you're fatigued.
Exercise and Physical Work	Moving your body.	Increases blood flow and electrical activity in muscles; entrains your muscles; entertains your mind; enhances motivation and lengthens time and distance performance.
Thrills	Looking for a rush or pleasure fix.	Gives physical and emotional thrills; excites your nervous system; stimulates your emotional response; activates your reward circuit through tension and release.

Music is audio fuel for action. When the sound of stimulating music hits your inner ear, your cochlea converts it into electrical energy and sends it into your brain. These electrical impulses travel through your cortex, down your spine, through the sinoatrial node (the pacemaker for your heart), and out into your muscles, arousing every element of your autonomic nervous system as they go. In short, the right kind of music literally electrifies your body.

Experiments using electroencephalograms to measure the arousal levels of people listening to Energizing music register increased heart rate, pulse, respiratory rate, and blood pressure, along with dilated pupils and greater galvanic skin response. Electromyograms measure increased electrical activity in muscles under music conditions. These are all signs of being awake and ready to act.[1]

Energizing music can also produce beta waves in your brain, the electrical patterns of about thirteen to thirty cycles per second that help you attend to external events, make quick decisions, and solve immediate problems.[2]

It may be a basic craving to be more awake in body and mind that makes people prefer music that moves at a faster speed with higher pitches and brighter sounds[3]—all characteristics of Energizing music. Everybody wants to feel up, and music is an effective and safe way to go.

Wake Up!

Your first cup of coffee in the morning makes you more alert than any others you drink during the day. After that, your body becomes accustomed to the caffeine and reacts less.[4] And so it is with sound. Your morning music can have greater impact on the rest of your waking cycle than anything else you hear during the day.

Holly, for instance, is not a morning person. She enjoyed her job as editor for a financial newsletter in New York because its late-night schedule suited her inner rhythms. Then she decided to switch directions and become a stock trader in San Francisco, where the market opens at six A.M.

Her first week on the job, Holly's new boss expressed concern about her slow start off the opening bell. Desperate for firepower to save her new job, Holly was soon drinking so much coffee that she couldn't sleep at night. She was fighting the shakes and worried about her health and her job when she stumbled on the solution: three minutes of loud rock and roll straight out of bed. A blast of the Rolling Stones or Pearl Jam helped her shower and dress faster and postponed the need for her first hit of caffeine until she got to work. Holly's morning music helped her recover her steady hands and sleeping habits—and brightened up the gray San Francisco dawn.

You might be surprised to learn that your circadian rhythms can be at their most vigorous when you first rise in the morning. That hazy hour when you stagger around with half-mast eyelids might actually be your physiological peak. But it often doesn't feel that way because your nervous system is still back in bed, trying to grab a few more minutes of sleep while you risk slitting your throat as you shave because your brain and hand aren't talking to each other yet.

The transition from the subconscious world to the conscious can be traumatic, but music can help. The world looks better when you wake up to a favorite tune, and, like that first cup of coffee, the energy benefits of early listening are at their peak.

Braintuning Basics: Wake Up!

....

Ear Coffee

For an easy and instant audio energizer:

- **First things first.** Have your music right out of bed, before the kids or pets come running or the morning paper calls. A jump start, by definition, has to happen at the beginning.

- **Cue up your selection the night before.** Planning is important because your sleepy morning head has a way of deciding it doesn't *need* that ear coffee. "Too much trouble!" whisper your nerves in a conspiracy to protect your slumbering synapses.

- To further simplify the process, **make a tape of your favorite morning songs** and listen to one each day.

- **Broadcast the sound through speakers.** Sending sound waves through the air allows them to surround your whole body for a live listening experience. Use headphones only if other people's sleep patterns require it.

- **Turn up the music as loud** as your family, neighbors, and good health allow.

- **Dance.** You might miss beats, but movement wakes up your muscles and metabolism. It appears that the same neural networks that encode music control your movement,[5] so moving to music in the morning tunes up your physical and mental coordination for the day and over the long term.

- **Keep it short and snappy.** Time is at a premium in the morning, so the three to four minutes of an average pop song should do.

- **Shine the light.** Energizing music is especially important if it's cold and dark when you get up. Stimulating sounds can simulate daylight to warm your body and mind.

Ear Care

If your music is too loud, you're not tuning your brain, you're chewing up your eardrums. Hearing loss is permanent and irrevocable. Your continued ability to enjoy the pleasures and benefits of sound depend upon a preventive approach to ear health, which includes carefully controlling the volume of all your listening experiences.

OSHA sets the safe level of sound over the course of an eight-hour day at ninety decibels[6] (by comparison, a vacuum cleaner averages about seventy-five decibels). Practical criteria for short-term listening is that when you're done, your ears shouldn't ring and your hearing should seem clear, not muted. Also remember that your ears adapt to higher volumes over time, so resist the urge to notch it up after listening for awhile. You should never wear headphones while driving or bicycling; they can block the sounds of traffic and sirens. Some safety experts recommend against using headphones while walking or running for the same reason, and add that women in particular should be alert to the sounds of potential assailants.

On a positive note, some recent evidence points to a very small correlation between exposure to music and risk of hearing damage.[7] But play it safe. No braintuning benefit is worth jeopardizing the acuity of your hearing.

Presentations and Performance

Once you've woken up, there remain parts of the day when you will need an extra hit of energy for high-powered performance. Alertness and positive thinking can make a critical difference whenever you have to perform—in a presentation, meeting, test, audition, interview, lecture, sales pitch, or any other situation involving an audience looking at or listening to *you*. But late nights preparing and last-minute nerves can often leave you feeling fatigued and empty just when you need to shine. When you want to put your best face forward, music can shift you into high gear.

Julie, head of marketing at a Web page design firm, straps on her Discman and struts around to James Brown's "I Feel Good" before every client presentation. She knows this helps her make an impression, but she might not know the details of how: The syncopated drum beat, high-pitched guitar riffs, horn punches, and famous James Brown shouts pull Julie out of the still and silent world of the Internet, stimulating her nervous system and parts of her brain that she needs for an effective presentation.

The musical massage of Julie's cortex gets her neurons firing to help her think fast. The wake-up of her cerebellum, the center of coordination, enhances her physical presence and enables her to flip screens and gesture with conviction. And her animated hypothalamus, home of instinctual response, gears up to give her the gut instinct she needs to get a commitment. With the last guitar chord ringing in her mind, Julie greets her potential client with all systems go.

Preparing for performance with energizing music gives you a triple edge. First, it operates physiologically to stimulate your system and sharpen your alertness, participation, and attentiveness.[8] Second, listening to music can deliver a burst of increased self-esteem, giving you the confidence you need to succeed.[9] And third, a self-programmed listening session takes you out of the sterile environment of an office or dressing room and colors your attitude with the dynamics of beat and sound.

Braintuning Basics: Presentations and Performance

High-Impact Listening

For the maximum musical boost before an appearance:

- **Pump up the volume.** Sound waves are energy, and higher volumes actually send more electrical pulses per second into your brain. Turn up the music until it resonates through every meridian of your body—but *never* listen to music at a level that causes pain or discomfort (see Ear Care on page 31). Feel the electricity enter your brain, speed along synapses, then move down your spinal cord and into your body, waking up nerves and muscles all the way to your fingers and toes.

- **Tweak the high end.** Upper frequencies penetrate directly to your arousal centers, so emphasize the music's high end with the tone control knob or equalizer of your stereo.

- **Pay attention.** Power listening is focused listening, and paying attention to energizing music arouses your system more. Make the music the total experience of the moment. Let the beat fill you up and move you from within.

- **Dance.** A body in motion is self-arousing. As you move to the rhythm of the music, the oxygen demands of your muscles speed your heart rate, breathing, and metabolism, while the entraining of your movements to the meter internalizes the stimulating beat. Even chair dancing will enhance the benefits of energizing music, so move what you can.

- **Change the pace.** If your listening session extends beyond a single piece of music, change styles from one selection to the next—from rock to symphonic music, from drum-heavy samba to the wailing drone of bagpipes. A variety of beats and sounds have been shown to have the greatest stimulative effect.[10]

- **Use headphones in other people's environments** to help you focus on preparing yourself. Exception: group performance.

- **Time precisely.** The closer your listening session is to your performance, the more effective it will be. The energizing benefits of music can fade with time, so have extra music on hand to fill unexpected delays, and keep your headphones on until the last possible minute.

Competition and Negotiations

There's awake, the maintenance level of arousal required for a productive day, and then there's **awake,** the alertness you need to make your way through struggles, stand-offs, sports, and power relations. Olympic Gold medalist Michael Johnson reported listening to jazz to gear up for the 400-meter race, but he needed the more aggressive sounds of gangsta rap to prepare him for his record-breaking 19.32-second performance on the 200-meter run.[11]

Most cultures use music to send their soldiers off to war. Engagements from the football field to the boardroom require extra energy and personal power, both of which can be conjured up by the right music. Use Energizing music to add confidence, clarity of purpose, even aggression to your next game, deal, or fight to save the rain forest.[12]

Braintuning Basics: Competition and Negotiations

- **Use focused listening** as soon before the engagement as possible to keep your energy fresh.

- **Choose music that means victory to you.** When a song helps you to succeed, use it again the next time to condition yourself to win.

- **Get the heartbeat edge.** Make sure you're thinking and moving faster than the competition by preparing with music faster than the resting human heartbeat. Songs that move at ninety-five beats per minute or more will get you up to speed.

- **Tune up with team listening.** If your encounter involves a group of people, as do many business deals or sporting events, bring along a portable tape player and listen together to create a group vibe.

Recharge

No matter how well you manage your energy, biorhythms dictate that you'll hit the wall every once in awhile. It's natural—but it's rarely convenient. The ubiquitous coffee break is a signpost of a society that likes to work long but sedentary days in which refreshing breaks are crucial to continued productivity. Your nervous system slows down after a few hours of sitting at your desk, and brain drain is often the result.

Curt, an insurance actuary, used to counter his daily three o'clock slump with Coke and a Snickers bar until he discovered the reviving power of Haydn's Military Symphony and a walk around the block. He's taken off ten pounds, and is thrilled to be in a lower risk group on the insurance tables.

Splashing some coffee, sugar, or a smart drink on your sleeping nerves is one way to return to the living, but wouldn't it be nicer to wake them up with a wash of energizing music?

Braintuning Basics: Recharge

Alertness Breaks

Quick, efficient, and cheaper than a latte:

- **Suit up.** Keep a Walkman or Discman in your desk and get it out when your brain begins to fog.

- **Cue up.** Choose a short, smart, energizing selection with plenty of volume. Keep a selection of discs or a special alertness-break tape at the office or in the car.

- **Make it strange.** Unfamiliar sounds create more neurological excitement than those you know, so take advantage of your suspicious mind to let new music wake up your brain cells.

- **Freshen up** with movement. It's best if you can slip outside for a walk while you listen. An alternative is to open a window and breathe the air; follow with a brisk stroll around the office.

- **Tune out** from your surroundings and lose yourself in the music. Part of the rejuvenating effect is in the break from your daily environment.

Musical Snacks

Coffee is only half the content of the classic coffee break. The other is the snack you might gulp down with little need for the calories. Food *seems* to present an easy solution to boredom and fatigue during the course of the working day, but most snack attacks are rooted in boredom and an instinctual urge to stimulate your metabolism, which can slow down with sedentary work and your natural circadian rhythms. Eating works, but the calories you consume more than compensate for any metabolic lift, so skip the doughnut and pick up your Discman for a three-minute musical snack. Experts agree that nutritious snacks in proper portions can be an important component of a healthy eating plan; use this braintuning strategy to address unhealthy or excessive eating behaviors. Add a dance, and you might even burn body fat.

Asleep at the Wheel

If anything can be more sleep-inducing than a day at work, it's driving down a long, open road. Drowsy driving may account for as many as 10,000 traffic fatalities a year in the United States alone. Studies show that 25 percent of all drivers have fallen asleep behind the wheel, resulting in crashes for one in ten of them.[13]

You can use Energizing music as a preventive strategy any time you drive, but here are sure signs that you need a recharge break:

- Your head nods or eyes droop.

- You feel lost or disoriented.

- You find yourself swerving or veering.

- Your reaction time slows.

If you experience any of these situations in the car, roll down the window and put on some Energizing music. Crank up the volume and sing along at the top of your lungs. If that doesn't work, get off the road immediately. The recharge you need is called sleep.

Exercise and Work

He who mingles music with gymnastic in the fairest proportions,
and best attempers them to the soul, may be rightly called
the true musician and harmonist in a far higher sense than
the tuner of the strings.

—Plato, Book IV of *The Republic*

Plato may have been the first proponent of aerobic dancing. Though he predated the age of health clubs with industrial-strength sound systems, Plato understood the natural connection between music and movement— the same link that makes a *sogo* drum in West Africa cause the dancer to shake like a leaf, or the funky groove in an aerobics class to motivate higher kicks and jumps. At the laboratories of the National Institutes of Health, it was found that people who practice the piano—or even *imagine it*—more than triple the size of the motor maps that control muscles and coordination in their brains,[14] while in the hospital, palsied patients who can't tap their toes when verbally instructed to do so start pounding away when the music begins.[15] In his book *Awakenings*, neurologist Oliver Sacks describes a patient essentially paralyzed by Parkinson's disease who regained motion, power, and control by replaying music in her mind.[16] And music theorist David Epstein proposes a biological basis for musical time in which the natural tempo of the body's movements guides a musician's performance speed.[17]

In fact, sound, particularly as it manifests in music, is the only human sense to represent time—and it turns out that muscle movements originate with timekeeping structures in the brain.[18] Physiologists and psychologists have confirmed the music-movement correlation, discovering in clinical trials that music improves mental attitude toward exercise and actual motor performance. One study showed that participants who listened to music walked a quarter mile farther in thirty minutes than those who didn't—*and* they showed a faster heart rate recovery afterward.[19] On the stationary bike, music has been found to increase mileage for both active and inactive adults and children, and on the treadmill, it boosts the respiratory rate of trained and untrained runners.[20] Using music as a reward during practice improved training behaviors among competitive swimmers and left them asking for more.[21] Music has long been used to facilitate movement in the ill, injured, or handicapped, and a recent study found that patients with lung disease exercised for 22 percent longer to music than to silence or gray noise, and worked 44 to 53 percent harder.[22]

Whether you run or Rollerblade, lift weights, bike, or box, Energizing music can make you exercise longer and harder. It increases speed and workload capacity for greater conditioning benefits, while it lowers perceived exertion rate. Listening to music while you move can hasten your post-exercise recovery. The aggregate of research shows that music with a strong, steady beat can:

- Increase endurance
- Boost effort level
- Regularize pace, gait, and breathing
- Enhance muscle control
- Increase motivation
- Distract from discomfort[23]

It's the autonomic nervous system that turns braintuning into bodytuning, and the process begins before you even start to move: Energizing music gently boosts your heart and respiratory rates to prepare you for the more intense effort that follows. This warm-up at the nervous system level improves your outlook, making you feel powerful and energized. As you begin to move, the music provides physiological entraining—rhythm—for your muscles, entertainment for your mind, and inspiration for the spirit of your efforts.

Exercise Good Ear Judgment

You should always be careful when you pump up the volume of Energizing music—but use extra caution if you're also pumping iron or anything else. It's possible that exercise makes your ears more vulnerable to temporary noise-induced threshold shifts in your hearing.[24] The noise level of many health clubs can also induce you to edge up the volume on your headphones farther than you normally would.

One aerobics instructor who surveyed his classes found that the minimum volume that made participants happy was 85 to 90 decibels—within the OSHA guidelines for daily exposure and well below the 105-decibel cap for one hour.[25] If you feel instructors are playing the music too loud, ask them to turn it down. Follow the guidelines at the beginning of this chapter and be as good to your ears as you are to the rest of your body.

Braintuning Basics: Exercise and Work

Electric Exercise

- **Prime the pump** by listening to Energizing music before you even begin to work out—in the car on your way to the basketball court or on a Discman as you wait for class to begin—for a motionless warm-up of your nervous and cardiovascular system.

- **Incorporate variety** into your workout music. Contrasts in style, beat, and texture—even intermittent periods of silence—enhance your exercise performance.[26] It seems your muscles wake up all over again when you move from rap to a trumpet concerto.

- **Suit yourself.** Music you like gives the best boost to your workout, while sounds that displease you might actually impede your exercise efforts.[27] Have you ever suddenly lost the desire to move when a song you hate came on? Or there's the disturbing tendency of class instructors to increase the tape speed and turn your favorite track into a Chipmunks song. It turns out that though people generally prefer their music faster and brighter, altering popular recordings from their original versions is clinically proven to turn people off.[28] Take control of your workout music by using your own tapes for solo activities and being a selective student in classes. Seek out instructors who play music appropriate to the activity, match their movement and yours to the rhythm, and share your musical tastes.

That's Entrainment

Want better coordination, greater endurance, deeper conditioning, and more regular breathing? You can *entrain* your muscles by matching the pace of your movement to the speed of your music. A study that measured arm muscle activity during a flexing and striking routine found that adding an audio rhythm track regularized the electrical impulses of the muscles, increased cocontraction of the biceps and triceps, and increased the duration of the muscles' effort. That's what we call entrainment.[29]

To use music to entrain your muscles and enhance the conditioning effect of your exercise:

- **Time your workout pace.** Watch the second hand and count your moves for one minute.

- **Time your music.** Count the beats you hear in a minute.

- **Match your music to your movement.** You can either look for a direct match of beats to moves (good for running, for example), or use a beats-per-minute count that's an even multiple of your moves per minute. For instance, many people who lift weights to music use four beats for the positive movement (lifting) and four beats for the negative (lowering). That's eight beats per rep, so if you typically do twelve reps per minute, use music that moves at 96 beats per minute (a typical tempo for hip hop).

- **To push your exercise speed,** choose music that's slightly faster than your current workout pace. **To push your intensity instead,** try music that's slightly slower than your normal speed.

- **Make several tapes** of a wide variety of styles that follow the pace of your workout, matching the tempo to your warm-up, each activity in your exercise session, and cool-down. Rotate your tapes often to prevent boredom.

Tempo, Tempo

Here are some ways to experiment with matching music from the Energize discography with your workout. You can explore further as you get a feel for the speed of your moves.

- **Heartbeat rate (70–90 beats per minute):** In an experiment where stationary bikers controlled the tempo of the music they heard with their pedaling speed, they preferred rates between 70 and 90 revolutions per minute.[30] Music at this heartbeat tempo can help you get started if you're feeling sluggish. Then you can work up from there.

    Example (beats per minute): Anita Baker, "Sweet Love" (86; from chapter 2, Relax)

- **Slow (90–120 beats per minute):** Weightlifting, weight machines, Stairmaster, stairs (walking), Versaclimber, rowing, Rollerblading, slow walking or hiking, floor exercises, cooling down, and stretching.

    Examples (beats per minute):
    Stevie Wonder, "Superstition" (100)
    Pearl Jam, "Jeremy" (106)
    Parliament, "Give Up the Funk (Tear the Roof Off the Sucker)" (106)
    Boston, "More Than a Feeling" (110)
    The Sugarhill Gang, "Rapper's Delight" (112)
    Nirvana, "Smells Like Teen Spirit" (116)
    Berlioz, "La Marseillaise" (116)
    Most hip hop

- **Midtempo (120–135 beats per minute):** Warming up,* power walking or hiking, treadmill, stairs (running), step or slide aerobics, interval training.

    Examples (beats per minute):
    The Temptations, "Ain't Too Proud to Beg" (120)
    Creedence Clearwater Revival, "Proud Mary" (120)
    Mickey Hart, "Udu Chant" (128, *The Big Bang*)

*Make sure your warm-up music really gets you going—something you like that provides a mental boost for the effort to follow.

The Doors, "Light My Fire" (128)

Sly & the Family Stone, "Dance to the Music" (128)

Howlin' Wolf, "Smokestack Lightnin' " (128)

Lina Santiago, "Feels So Good" (130)

The Clash, "London Calling" (134)

The Catelli All Stars, "Do Back Back" (134, *Heart of Steel*)

MC Hammer, "U Can't Touch This" (134)

Most house and techno

- **Fast (135+ beats per minute):** Jogging, bicycling, aerobics.
  Examples (beats per minute):

  Booker T & the MGs, "Green Onions" (136)

  Michael Jackson, "Beat It" (138)

  The Eagles, "Take It Easy" (138)

  Elvis Costello, "Pump It Up" (140)

  Offenbach, 4th Allegro on *Gaite Parisienne* (150)

  Lynyrd Skynyrd, "Free Bird" (152, fast part; warm up to the first 6 minutes)

  Chuck Berry, "Johnny B. Goode" (170)

  Led Zeppelin, "Rock and Roll" (170)

  Elvis Presley, "Jailhouse Rock" (172)

  The Ramones, "Sheena Is a Punk Rocker" (178)

Always choose a speed that enables a full range of motion for whatever you're doing. For efficient muscle work and fat-burning, you might want to cap your workout pace at 140 moves per minute. You can work to faster music—just move with every two or four beats. Conversely, you can use down-tempo music like hip-hop and work twice as fast as the beat. What matters is not how many beats each movement takes but that you move in synch with the rhythm you hear.

Attitude Adjustment

Adding music to exercise has an even more positive effect on the attitudes of untrained minds and bodies than on conditioned athletes, so if you're just starting out, or the very idea of exercise runs against the grain of your personality, let music help you decide to just do it.

Work

Though it's increasingly rare in our sedentary society, sometimes you move your body to actually get something done. The positive link between music and movement isn't limited to people in Spandex; it also holds for physical work like raking leaves, washing windows, or building houses. When constructing the ancient Theban city of Messene, Epaminoadas asked musicians to accompany the labor to make it go easier. Traditional folk musics includes work songs to accompany tasks from picking olives to mining coal to cooking; in Japan, for instance, the recorded history of agricultural work songs goes back over 1,000 years. You can get the same motivational, endurance, and entraining benefits from music in the garden or at the construction site as in the gym, so take advantage of Energizing music any time you move.

Thrills

Thrills: the lighter side of energizing. You get them climbing mountains, bungee jumping, at adventure movies, in erotic embrace—and while listening to music. In fact, the existence of musical rush has been acknowledged for centuries. The Arabs call it *tarab*—the unique state of ecstasy brought on only by music. In Middle Eastern culture, music performances are often accompanied by ecstatic moans from the audience.

The physiology of thrills is still only partly understood. However, one test measuring the thrills that people experience listening to music came to the titillating conclusion that music can cause "chills, shudders, tingling, and tickling" in the upper spine, back of the neck, shoulders, lower spine, and scalp. These feelings can then radiate outward to the shoulders and arms and travel the length of your spine. And, yes, they're even known to sweep across the chest, genitals, thighs, and legs.[31] Not bad for an earful of sound with no potentially injurious outcomes.

Even better, it turns out that music was the stimulus most frequently reported to create thrills, beating out sex, sports, and beautiful paintings and sculptures. The experimenter postulates that musical thrills might result from spreading electrical activity in the brain, extending through neural links to the limbic and autonomic nervous systems. Another study found that the opiate-blocking drug Naloxene significantly reduced the pleasure that people experienced while listening to music, suggesting that music might actually produce endorphins—pleasure chemicals—in the brain.[32]

Part of music's thrill factor lies in its juxtaposition of tension and release. In many classical compositions, the pattern of buildup and delivery is structured into sonata form, which states a theme, develops and transforms it, then restates it with a climactic twist. Music theorist Anthony Storr likens this organization to that of archetypal hero myths and modern novels.[33] Psychologist Leonard Meyer goes a step further by describing classical music structure as a process of creating expectations, postponing their fulfillment, then finally providing the goods in a great climactic moment.[34] Sound like any other exciting activity you know?

An experimenter who tested people's sexual arousal while listening to classical music found that the better people liked the music they heard, the more it turned them on.[35] The study also discovered that music-induced sexual arousal was strongest among anxious, introverted people, suggesting that the private, controlled nature of musical thrills is particularly attractive when you're less likely to engage in more extroverted activities.

For more about using music to add impetus to your sex life, see chapter 7, Create.

Impulses and Addictions

The natural human need for thrills lies behind recreations as diverse as mountain biking and crack cocaine. Unrestrained thrill-seeking can lead to impulsive behavior—a shopping spree, unplanned weekend trip, or impromptu drag race. If your impulses hit harder, you might opt for an alcohol or drug binge, or a high-stakes run at the craps table. In any case, the goal of such behavior is an instant escape from daily life, inner demons, or feelings of emptiness.

When the need for stimulation is strong and constant, it becomes an impulse control disorder. Some psychologists describe the inability to control impulses as "reward deficiency syndrome," in which brain pathways fail to deliver adequate satisfaction messages. The result can be sensation-seeking behavior, cravings, and the need for immediate gratification—drives that in the extreme have been linked to alcoholism; drug addiction; binge eating and bulimia; compulsive gambling, buying, and smoking; kleptomania; and self-mutilative behavior.[36]

Psychiatrists first got the idea of treating impulsive behavior with music in the early nineteenth century, 150 years before music therapy moved into the mainstream. It was Dr. Edwin Atlee who proposed using music to cure what was then called mania: "the consequences of a delirious or mistaken idea."[37]

When you want to control your own cravings for a hot fudge sundae, a double Scotch, or a hundred dollar bet on the football game, look for immediate gratification from music instead.

Braintuning Basics: Thrills

Have an Eargasm

The sexually tinged tension-climax-release pattern of music—especially Western classical compositions—is so broadly accepted that it's even been the subject of feminist deconstructionism.[38] To take advantage of this no-strings-attached erotic thrill:

- Pick music with clearly discernible climaxes (try selections from the Thrills section of the discography).

- As the musical tension mounts, try to put the feeling into your body: muscles, nerves, erogenous zones.

- Hear and feel the approach of the climax. Work for it, wish for it, live for it.

- When the big crash comes, feel it as a physical explosion, then relax into the sweet sounds of release.

The Energizing Music-Mood Checklist

- ❑ Quick tempo, 95 beats per minute or more
- ❑ Lively, loud, emphatic beat
- ❑ Syncopated, compound, dotted, or ragged rhythms
- ❑ Percussive or staccato feeling
- ❑ Large ensembles
- ❑ Full sound
- ❑ Loud volume
- ❑ Bright, brash tone colors
- ❑ Surprising or unexpected sounds

❑ High pitches

❑ Large tonal range

Avoid dragging beats, slow or medium tempos, bass-heavy sounds, thin textures, and sad tunes or harmonies.[39]

Test Your Musical Juice

See page 24 in the introduction for instructions on testing your music-mood response. An Energize discography follows the quiz. Start by testing your favorite styles from the list and recording your results in the journal that follows.

The Energize Music-Mood Test

I Feel	Before Listening (1–5)	After Listening (1–5)	Change, Before to After (+ or −, 0–4)
Awake	_____	_____	_____
Quick	_____	_____	_____
Inspired	_____	_____	_____
Vivacious	_____	_____	_____
Motivated	_____	_____	_____
Active	_____	_____	_____
Talkative	_____	_____	_____
Attentive	_____	_____	_____
Powerful	_____	_____	_____
Excited	_____	_____	_____

Total Change:
Your Energy Response (0–40) _____

The Energize Music-Mood Journal

Date	Situation	Selection	Score
_____	_____	_____	_____
_____	_____	_____	_____
_____	_____	_____	_____
_____	_____	_____	_____
_____	_____	_____	_____
_____	_____	_____	_____
_____	_____	_____	_____
_____	_____	_____	_____
_____	_____	_____	_____
_____	_____	_____	_____
_____	_____	_____	_____
_____	_____	_____	_____
_____	_____	_____	_____
_____	_____	_____	_____
_____	_____	_____	_____
_____	_____	_____	_____
_____	_____	_____	_____
_____	_____	_____	_____
_____	_____	_____	_____

Braintuning Music: Energize

The Energize discography encompasses the brisk, bright, rhythmic music that stimulates mental and physical sharpness. Think of the military marches used to rally soldiers for battle; the big samba drum ensembles that accompany all-night Carnival parades in Rio; or the driving beats of rock and rap that are credited with propelling ecstatic dance parties or accused of stimulating dangerously aggressive behavior, depending upon whom you talk to. Energizing music is made mostly of beat and speed.

Another characteristic of Energizing music is the element of surprise. Unfamiliar music can generate more neurological and physical arousal than the tried and true—so this is a good time to explore new sounds.

On the other hand, you can also condition yourself to associate certain familiar songs or styles with getting psyched. Whether you choose the known or the new, listen for sounds that leap up out of the groove.

Drums

Energy begins with the big bang of the drum, which pounds with the primeval heartbeat that powers human life. Long used to make people move and forming the basis of most Energizing music, drums tap your internal rhythms and drive them forward.

For an unadulterated dose of drums, try percussion traditions like African drum ensembles, Japan's athletic **taiko** groups, or the beats of Middle Eastern belly dancing.

Many of the most rhythmic musical styles in the New World derive from African drumming. Afro-Cuban **rumba** adds call-and-response vocals to a mix of African percussion, while **salsa** and **Latin jazz** blend Latin dance forms and American jazz—hot sauce for the ears.

In Brazil, percussion, *berimbau* (a bow that resonates on the human body), and vocals accompany the martial art and dance called **capoeira**. **Samba** is the soundtrack to the endless revelries of Carnival, and its *bateria* of big drums will bring you back to life no matter how long you've been dead. Or maybe you prefer to steel your nerves with the sound of tuned oil drums—"pan," or **steel band** music from Trinidad and Tobago. Originally formed for the street parades of Carnival, pan bands can include up to 2,000 steel drums in a moving wall of sound.

Rock, Rap, Soul and Funk

Perhaps the quintessential performance music is **your favorite rock, rap, soul, or funk song**. Whether it's "Satisfaction," "I Feel Good," or "Fight the

Power," favorite jams have powered students into exams and surgeons into the O/R for decades. You don't have to give up this habit because you've made VP—just be sure you have a pair of well-insulated headphones. The Rock and Roll Hall of Fame has named "500 Songs that Shaped Rock and Roll," and a selection of the most Energizing tunes is listed in the discography.

Horns

The sound of the horn has woken people up and sent them off to combat for centuries. If you've been to Scout camp, you know a trumpet reveille can rouse you whether you like it or not. In the **classical orchestra**, the brass section offers fanfares, calls, and flourishes to snap you to attention and summon up your beta waves. Many of the classical selections in the Energize discography feature horns, front and center.

Brass bands usually specialize in marches, which are specially designed to make you move. A Philadelphia radio station wakes its morning commute listeners with a "Sousalarm" every day—a Sousa march to clear foggy minds before the workday begins.

Jazz is known for pushing the upper limits of the trumpet's range. High-horn pioneers like Dizzy Gillespie and Roy Eldridge can clear your sinuses with very exciting frequencies.

Like a horn but not quite: **bagpipes.** The untempered tuning of bagpipes gives them an otherworldly sound, and because all the notes are in the harmonic overtone series, they truly resonate in your body. One piper said that bagpipes "awaken the genetic memory of those of us with even a smidgen of Celtic blood"; another reported that he celebrates successes by playing the "Ode to Joy" on bagpipes. Long associated with outdoor celebrations and the military, pipes will prepare you to cut a jig or fight like Rob Roy.

Disco, Dance & Techno

Not only are dance grooves meant to make you move, but their popularity in health clubs might have your mind and muscles conditioned to spring into action with the first thud of the bass drum. Some dance selections are listed here; for a world of dance music, refer also to the discography in chapter 5, Uplift.

Thrills

When you want more than just bang for your buck . . . When you seek the high of delayed gratification and subsequent release . . . When you crave a musical thrill, these are the selections to try. Music theorist Terence Mc-Laughlin has identified what he calls "the erotic phrase" in certain classical works,[40] and many pieces built on the aesthetic base of tension and resolution can send a tingle down your spine—or wherever you want it to go.

The Braintuning Discography: Energize

STYLE	TITLE
Drums	• *The Big Bang*. Ellipsis Arts 3400. 3 CDs guaranteed to make you groove all the way from Cuba to Japan. Make a tape of the most motivating tracks to prepare for big meetings and games. • R.A. Fish. *Rhythmic Essence: The Art of the Dumbek*. Lyrichord 7411. Belly dancing beats on the classic Middle Eastern drum. • Mickey Hart. *Planet Drum*. Rykodisc 10206. A global groove tour compiled by Mickey Hart of the Grateful Dead. • Babatunde Olatunji. *Drums of Passion: The Beat*. Rykodisc 10107. From West Africa. • Cornel Pewardy & the Alliance West Singers. "Buffalo Dances," "Kiowa Gourd Dance Songs," "Hethuska War Dance Song," "War Dance Songs," "Horse Stealing and Trot Songs," and "War Journey Songs" on *Dancing Buffalo*. Music of the World 130. Authentic Native American drumming and singing from peoples of the Southern Plains; try it before your next horse-stealing raid. • *Soh Daiko*. Lyrichord 7410. Japanese *taiko* drumming uses an ensemble of big drums played with split-second choreography. Shinto belief holds that *taiko* communicates with the gods and mobilizes warring armies. • *Songs of Earth, Water, Fire and Sky: Music of the American Indian*. New World 80246. Try the Seneca Alligator Dance or the Southern Plains people's Oklahoma Two-Step.
Rumba Salsa	• Los Muñequitos de Matanzas. *Cantar Maravilloso*. Globestyle 053. Celia Cruz. *The Best*. Sony Discos 80587. • *The Mambo Kings Soundtrack*. Elektra 961240. Celia Cruz, Tito Puente, and Arturo Sandoval.
Latin Jazz	• Eddie Palmieri. *Lucumi Macumba Voodoo—Legendas*. Sony Discos 81530. • Arturo Sandoval. *Danzon (Dance On)*. GRP 9761. Leading trumpeter in Afro-Cuban session with guest appearance by Gloria Estefan.

Capoeira	• *Capoeira Angola from Salvador, Brazil*. Smithsonian Folkways 40645.
Samba	• *Brazil Classics II: O Samba*. Sire 26019. • DJ Dero. *Volumen 1*. Oid Mortales/BMG 30222. In "Batucada," the Argentinian DJ brings samba to the dance floor with *batería* drums like sonic rocket fuel.
Steel Band	• Steelbands of Trinidad and Tobago. *The Heart of Steel*. Flying Fish 70522. Take pieces like Offenbach's "Orpheus in the Underworld," perform them with huge ensembles of tuned steel drums and plenty of percussion—and you're as awake as you care to be. • Our Boys Steel Orchestra. *Pan Progress*. Mango 539916.
Rock & Roll Hall of Fame	• AC/DC. "Back in Black" on *Back in Black*. Atlantic 92418. • Chuck Berry. "Johnny B. Goode," "Maybellene," and "Rock & Roll Music" on *Chuck Berry: The Great Twenty-Eight*. Chess/MCA 92500. • Booker T and the MGs. "Green Onions" on *Top of the Stax: Twenty Greatest Hits*. Stax 88005. • Kurtis Blow. "The Breaks" on *Best of Kurtis Blow*. Mercury 22456. • Boston. "More Than a Feeling" on *Boston*. Epic 34188. • James Brown. "I Got You (I Feel Good)" on *20 All Time Greatest Hits*. Polydor 511326. • The Clash. "London Calling" on *London Calling*. Epic 36328. • Elvis Costello. "Pump It Up" on *This Year's Model*. Rykodisc 10272. • Creedence Clearwater Revival. "Fortunate Son," "Green River," and "Proud Mary" on *Chronicle: 20 Greatest Hits*. Fantasy CCR-2. • De La Soul. "Me Myself & I" on *Me Myself & I*. Tommy Boy 926. • The Doors. "Light My Fire" on *Best of the Doors*. Elektra 60345. • The Eagles. "Take It Easy" on *Their Greatest Hits*. Asylum 253017. • Aretha Franklin. "Respect" on *30 Greatest Hits*. Atlantic 81668. • Jimi Hendrix. "Purple Haze." on *Are You Experienced?* MCA 10893. • Howlin' Wolf. "Smokestack Lightnin' " on *Chess Blues Classics*, 1947–1956. MCA/Chess 9369. • Michael Jackson. "Beat It" on *Thriller*. Epic 38112.

• Joan Jett. "I Love Rock & Roll" on *I Love Rock & Roll*. Blackheart 747.

• The Kinks. "You Really Got Me" on *Greatest Hits, Vol. 1*. Rhino 70086.

• Kiss. "Rock & Roll All Night" on *Alive!*. Casablanca 822780.

• Led Zeppelin. "Rock & Roll" on *Led Zeppelin IV*. Atlantic 82638.

• Jerry Lee Lewis. "Great Balls of Fire" on *18 Original Sun Greatest Hits*. Rhino 70255.

• Little Feat. "Dixie Chicken" on *Dixie Chicken*. Warner Brothers 2686.

• Lynyrd Skynyrd. "Free Bird" on *Gold & Platinum*. MCA 6898. The fast part.

• MC Hammer. "U Can't Touch This" on *Please Hammer Don't Hurt 'Em*. Capitol 92857.

• Nirvana. "Smells Like Teen Spirit" on *Nevermind*. Geffen 24425.

• Parliament. "Give Up the Funk (Tear the Roof off the Sucker)" on *The Best of Parliament: Give Up the Funk*. Casablanca 526995.

• Pearl Jam. "Jeremy" on *Ten*. Epic 47857.

• Elvis Presley. "Jailhouse Rock" on *Top Ten Hits*. RCA 56383.

• Public Enemy. "Fight the Power" on *Fear of a Black Planet*. Def Jam 523446.

• The Ramones. "Sheena Is a Punk Rocker" on *Ramones Mania*. Sire 25709.

• Otis Redding. "Try a Little Tenderness" on *The Very Best of Otis Redding*. Rhino 71147.

• The Rolling Stones. "(I Can't Get No) Satisfaction" on *Big Hits, Vol. 1 (High Tide & Green Grass)*. ABKCO 8001.

• The Sex Pistols. "Anarchy in the U.K." on *Never Mind the Bollocks, Here's the Sex Pistols*. Warner Brothers 3147.

• Sly & the Family Stone. "Dance to the Music" on *Greatest Hits*. Epic 30325.

• Bruce Springsteen. "Born to Run" on *Born to Run*. Columbia 33795.

• The Staple Singers. "Respect Yourself" on *Top of the Stax: Twenty Greatest Hits*. Stax 88005.

• The Temptations. "Ain't Too Proud to Beg" on *All the Million Sellers*. Motown 5212.

• The Troggs. "Wild Thing" on *Best of the Troggs*. Polygram 22841.

• U2. "Sunday Bloody Sunday." *War*. Island 811148.

• Van Halen. "Jump" on *1984*. Warner Brothers 23985.

- The Who. "My Generation" on *Greatest Hits*. MCA 1496.
- Stevie Wonder. "Superstition" on *Original Musiquarium I*. Motown 6002.
- ZZ Top. "Legs" on *Eliminator*. Warner Brothers 23774.
- Or your own favorite jam.

Classical

- *Baroque Music for Trumpets*. Wynton Marsalis, Raymond Leppard & the English Chamber Orchestra. CBS Masterworks 42478. High-horn concertos and sonatas by Vivaldi, Telemann, and Pachelbel.
- Ludwig van Beethoven. Final movement on *Symphony No. 5*. Carlos Kleiber & the Vienna Philharmonic, Deutsche Grammophon 447400. Heroic trumpets and Beethoven's renowned full sound.
- Hector Berlioz. "La Marseillaise," "Trojan March," and Rákóczy March" on *La Marseillaise & Other Berlioz Favorites*. David Zinman & the Baltimore Symphony Orchestra & Chorus, Telarc 80164. Crank up the French anthem and remember the rousing scene from "Casablanca."
- Georges Bizet. "March of the Toreadors" from *Carmen*. Sir Georg Solti, London Philharmonic, London 414489. Fast and crashing; good prep for a fight in the bullpen.
- George Friederic Handel. Alla Hornpipe, Movement 2 from Suite No. 2 in D Major. On *3 Suites ("Water Music"), HWV 348-350*, Archiv 410525. The brass fanfare is like a breath of fresh air.
- Franz Joseph Haydn. *Military Symphony No. 100*. RCA Victor 62564. The bright trumpet call to arms of this classical-era work was considered somewhat shocking—and was therefore quite popular—in 18th-century London.
- Gustav Holst. "Mars, the Bringer of War" on *The Planets*. James Levine & the Chicago Symphony Orchestra. Thick, clashing horns and pulsing motifs in the orchestra prepare you for your own personal battles.
- Aram Khatchaturian, "Sabre Dance" from *Gayane Suite*. Naxos 550800.
- Wolfgang Amadeus Mozart. First movement of *Symphony No. 35* and *Symphony No. 40*; first and final movement of *Symphony No. 41* on *Symphonies Nos. 35-41*. Karl Böhm & the Berlin Philharmonic, Deutsche Grammophon 447416. Combine string flourishes, horn calls, and timpani thunder for some elegant Energizers.
- Jacques Offenbach. Fourth allegro on *Gaite Parisienne*. Erich Kunzel & the Cincinnati Pops, Telarc 80294. Better known as the can-can.

• Maurice Ravel. "Bolero" on *Daphne et Chloe Suite No. 2*. Paul Paray & the Detroit Symphony Orchestra, Mercury Living Presence 34306. It might start slowly—but the martial beat and blaring horn are much better suited to a battle than the bedroom.

• Gioacchino Rossini. "William Tell Overture" on *Overtures*. Leonard Bernstein & the New York Philharmonic, Sony Classical 46713. The disc contains other rousing overtures such as Dvorak's *Carnival*, Offenbach's *Orpheus in the Underworld*, and more.

• Dmitri Shostakovich. Second and third movement of *Symphony No. 6*. Neemi Jarvi & the Scottish National Orchestra, Chandos 8411. From blaring horns and bassoon calls to a syncopated scherzo, this pair works together or alone.

• Peter Ilyich Tchaikovsky. *1812 Overture* and "Russian Dance" from *Nutcracker Suite*. London 417300. The cannons at the end of the 1812 are your signal to go to work.

• Giuseppe Verdi. "Grand March," *Aida*. Sir George Solti and the Rome Opera Orchestra and Chorus, London 417416.

• Richard Wagner. "Ride of the Valkyries" on *Richard Wagner*. Daniel Barenboim & the Orchestre de Paris, Deutsche Grammophon 445571. This famous number's horn call and stratospheric singing make a good warm-up for any wild ride.

• *Great Classical Marches*. Laserlight 15510. Works by Beethoven, Berlioz, Liszt and more.

Brass Bands

• The Dirty Dozen Brass Band. *New Orleans Album*. Columbia 45414.

• John Philip Sousa. *Original All-American Sousa*. Delos 3102. Sound your own Sousalarm with the original American marchmaster.

Bagpipes

• *The Bagpipe*. Lyrichord 7327. Marches, jigs, reels, and more from the whole Celtic family: Irish Uillean pipes, the *biniou* from Brittany, Galician *gaita*, and Scottish Highland bagpipes.

• Black 47. *Home of the Brave*. Chrysalis 30737. Celtic music gets truly loud with the addition of rock and roll and an impassioned Irish-New York sensibility.

• Forty-Eighth Highlanders. *Amazing Grace: Bagpipe Favorites*. Pro Arte 455.

Jazz

• Roy Eldridge. *After You've Gone*. Decca 605. This jazz master hit the high notes a generation before Dizzy.

• Dizzy Gillespie. *Dizzy's Diamonds: The Best of the Verve Years*. Verve 513875. Try the Afro-Cuban and big band tracks.

Disco, Dance, Techno

• Chemical Brothers. *Exit Planet Dust*. Astralwerks 6157. Acid house techno.

• Chic. *The Best of Chic: Dance, Dance, Dance*. Atlantic 82333.

• KC & the Sunshine Band. *The Best of KC & the Sunshine Band*. Rhino 70940.

• Chaka Khan. *Epiphany: The Best of Chaka Khan, Volume 1*. Reprise 45865.

• Madonna. *The Immaculate Collection*. Sire 26440. The dance diva's greatest hits.

• Prodigy. *Music for the Jilted Generation*. Mute/A.D.A. 9003. Hardcore techno.

• Quad City DJs. *Quad City DJs*. Atlantic 82905. "Tootsee Roll" and other dance floor favorites.

• Diana Ross. *Diana Extended—The Remixes*. Motown 6377.

• Lina Santiago. *Feels So Good*. MCA/Universal UD-53008. Latin dance music with a little house and hip-hop in the mix.

• *Start the Party! The Ultimate Collection of House Music*. Atlantic 92425.

• Donna Summer. *Donna Summer Anthology*. Casablanca 518144.

Thrills

• Carreras, Domingo & Pavarotti. *The Original Three Tenors in Concert*. Zubin Mehta, London 430433. The concert that started the three tenors craze. The energy level is as high as the macho competition is fierce.

• George Gershwin. *Rhapsody in Blue*. Neville Marriner & the Philharmonic Orchestra, Philips 411123.

• Wolfgang Amadeus Mozart. Zerlina's aria in *Don Giovanni*. John Eliot Gardiner, the English Baroque Soloists, and the Monteverdi Choir, Archiv 445870.

• Giaocchino Rossini. *Rossini Arias*. Cecilia Bartoli, Giuseppe Patané and the Konzertvereinigung Wiener Volksoperorchester, London 425430.

• Peter Ilyitch Tchaikovsky. *Romeo & Juliet Fantasy Overture in B Minor*. Herbert von Karajan & the Berlin Philharmonic, Deutsche Grammophon 439021.

• Second movement of *Symphony #5 in E Minor Op. 64*. Delos 3015.

• Richard Wagner. Prelude and Liebestod of *Tristan und Isolde* on *Richard Wagner*. Daniel Barenboim & the Orchestre de Paris, Deutsche Grammophon 445571.

See Page 255 for Sources.

Energize: The Braintuning 5

A diverse sampling from the discography to get you started:

The Big Bang. Ellipsis Arts 3400.

James Brown. *20 All Time Greatest Hits.* Polydor 511326.

Arturo Sandoval. *Danzon (Dance On).* GRP 9761.

Richard Wagner. Daniel Barenboim & the Orchestre de Paris, Deutsche Grammophon 445571.

Chic. *The Best of Chic: Dance, Dance, Dance.* Atlantic 82333.

Pump Up the Volume

From your first waking moment to your last late-night party, music can energize and electrify your every effort. In our Muzak society, much of the music you hear is designed to make you more passive. Don't fall for it when you need energy. Instead, pump up the volume to maximize your personal power and your joy in being awake and alive.

Two

Relax

We live in an age of high anxiety. Technology, the environment, and people in power seem to throw us a new curve every day. When stress puts you on edge, music can smooth you out, slow you down, and save you from the ravages of tension.

Relax Overview

Relaxing Music Can Help You With:	Use These Techniques if You Are:	How Music Helps:
Stress and Anxiety	Worried, nervous, jittery, overworked, on edge.	Slows your autonomic nervous system; enhances alpha brain wave production for clearer, calmer thought.
Patience	Stuck in traffic or a bank line, rushed and running behind, eating too fast.	Changes your perception of time to make it seem to pass more slowly.
People	Dealing with a difficult discussion or person.	Promotes conversation, communication, and a sense of shared well-being.

Panic	Prone to panic attacks.	Interrupts the trigger-panic cycle.
Balance	Seeking equilibrium between your outer and inner world.	Harmonizes the electrical impulses within your mind and body with the sound waves in the air of the outer world; activates your right brain to give the overworked logical left a break.
Meditation	Traveling to the world beyond conscious thought.	Fills your mind to push thoughts away; induces trance.
Sleep	Experiencing occasional or recurrent insomnia.	Slows heart rate, pulse, and breathing; shifts brain waves to delta patterns.

Most people like to relax to music, but have you ever wondered why Pearl Jam doesn't give you quite the same full-body meltdown as a bottle of Corona? The biological truth is that while your favorite tunes might seem like a good way to unwind, certain kinds of music bring the message home to your central nervous system better than others.[1] It takes the right sound waves to deliver the reliable neurophysiological slowdown of a stiff drink.

In a world where stress is the national standard and relaxation can be rare, learning to cool down with music can enhance and possibly even extend your life. Relaxing music flows through your nervous system to counteract the effects of stress on your body, while in your mind, the right kinds of music can stimulate alpha brain waves for clear thinking and patience, or the delta waves that signal sleep. When tension gets the upper hand and panic sets in, music can interrupt the negative biofeedback loop between the mind and body and give you some room to breathe. And on the interpersonal front, Relaxing music has been shown to promote communication among people, easing difficult discussions and averting potential confrontations. The techniques in this chapter will help you to use music as an agent of peace—in your mind, body, and relationships.

Stress and Anxiety

Stress is one of the most widespread and debilitating diseases in the United States. Whether your flash points are external stressors like traffic or deadlines, or internal feelings such as chronic tension or anxiety, you're probably familiar with the autonomic arousal signals stimulated by stress. In the face of perceived danger, your nervous system can raise your blood pressure, tense your muscles, and shorten your breath. Meanwhile, your endocrine system kicks in by releasing stress hormones like adrenaline and cortisol, which also happen to devour the immune cells that protect you against colds, flu, and other illness. Your physical meltdown is made worse by an implosion in your mind: anxiety, bad moods, poor concentration, and crumbling self-esteem. The price of all this activity can range from headaches and fatigue to increased risk of heart attack and stroke. Though its evolutionary purpose was to save your life by preparing you to fight or flee, stress in its modern manifestation is often an unwelcome attack upon your mind and body.

Fortunately, music can help manage your daily stress. Consider the case of Shelley, who works as an assistant for one of Hollywood's notorious screaming agents. Her first week on the job brought pounding headaches, acid stomach, and insomnia. To face the second Monday, Shelley decided she needed help.

She found it in a portable cassette player, which she brought to work, put on her desk, and used to soothe herself with music while she worked.

"Ambient dub saved my life—and my job," says Shelley. "If I'm listening to Orb I can stay cool while three phones ring, my boss screams, and I run the week's grosses. I lost my last job by screaming back. Now I close my mouth and let the music wash over me until I'm breathing again."

Shelley's instinct to treat her tension with music has its scientific base in medical research. A large body of clinical evidence shows that music can counteract stress on both physical and psychological levels. It can slow your pulse, heart rate, and breathing, lower your blood pressure, and relax your muscles.[2] Does anxiety have you literally gripping the edge of your seat? Relaxing music has been shown to loosen you up so much that it actually weakens the strength of your grip.[3] And it can reduce levels of the stress hormones in your blood that lead to fatigue and illness.[4]

Listening to the right music has also been shown to reduce general and task-related anxiety while triggering increased alpha wave activity in the brain, both of which bring the added bonus of enhanced concentration. From studies where background music boosted test scores in students with high test anxiety, to others linking music to improved performance by surgeons under stress, music has been shown to induce not only physical relaxation but also mental clarity.[5]

Anatomy of Anxiety

Anxiety is both a physiological and emotional state. During the 1960s, psychologist R. S. Lazarus was the first to propose that what we call anxiety is a combination of subjective feelings and autonomic nervous system arousal. Here are some of its signs.[6]

Physiological:

• Elevated heart rate

• Higher blood pressure

• Faster breathing

• Faster metabolism

• Constricted blood vessels

Behavioral:

• Restlessness

• Trembling

• Shortness of breath

• Muscular tension

• Fearful facial expressions

• Loss of appetite

• Fatigue

Relaxing music works at both the autonomic and emotional level to alleviate anxiety—before it reaches the cognitive plane and becomes worry.

In our breathless, frantic society, stress has earned the kind of notoriety usually reserved for incurable diseases, and perhaps with good reason. Stress is a prime culprit in heart disease, high blood pressure, digestive disorders, depressed immunity, fatigue, and burnout. Music can help you fight this public enemy—a personalized solution to a high-impact world.

Braintuning Basics: Stress and Anxiety

Loosen Up and Listen

In one experiment, listening to classical music lowered subjects' heart rates from an average of seventy-three beats per minute to seventy, but pop music sped them up from seventy-four to seventy-six,[7] so select your Relaxing music carefully and enhance its effects with the following techniques:

- **Go for a steady groove.** Changes in speed, volume, or overall sound can spark attention signals in your mind that interfere with the relaxation process, so avoid too much variety during any listening session.

- **Stick with the familiar.** Music is shown to get more relaxing with repeated listening.[8] Take advantage of the repetition effect by developing your own repertoire of favorite and familiar music to unwind with.

- **Program your CD player or make your own tapes.** Many compositions or CDs are sequenced for contrast, interspersing upbeat tracks with downtempo ones. An unexpected energizer will break your relaxed mood, so find the slow selections on each recording and stick to them when you want to unwind.

- **Use the iso principle** for gradual relaxation. Mood induction has been shown to be the most effective when you start with music that matches your current mood, then gradually move toward the state you want to attain.[9] Ease the transition to relaxation by beginning with music that corresponds to your present energy level, then making each selection slower, lower, and less intense than the one before.

- **Moderate the volume.** Loud music generates too much electrical energy to slow down your busy mind and body. Keep it soft enough for inner quiet, but just loud enough to surround you with tranquilizing sound.

- **Boost the bottom end** to make the sound richer and more comforting. Low frequencies calm you down the most, but you don't want booming bass. (Hint: if your bass booms, you've probably chosen the wrong sort of music for relaxation anyway.)

- **Get comfortable.** Whether you're taking a stress break at your desk with headphones and a portable player or lying on the living room floor between two stereo speakers, sit back or lie down as comfortably as you can.

- **Background listening: let it flow.** If you're listening to relaxing music in the background—at work, or during a meal or conversation—use a two-sided tape or multiple CDs so you won't have to hop up to change it. Then simply let the sound become a part of the air around you, keeping you calm and centered.

The Iso Principle at Play

Here's an example of how you can sequence a gradual relaxation session using the iso principle and selections from the discography in this chapter:

1. Anita Baker, "Sweet Love" (*Rapture*). At eighty-six beats per minute, this pop selection is on the upper end of the typical heart rate range, and has a strong drum beat, full production, and rich timbre to engage you at your normal operating level. (You may remember seeing it listed in the heartbeat range in the previous chapter.) Meanwhile, Baker's low voice and the familiar harmonies and song structure prepare you to move to the next level.

2. Zoot Sims, "You Go to My Head" (*For Lady Day*). Though this classic jazz tune is slightly faster (ninety beats per minute) than the previous selection, you're not likely to perceive it that way because the texture and pitch both take a dive down the curve toward relaxation. Tenor sax at the bottom of its range, understated piano and bass, and just a suggestion of brushed high hat and drums all notch down the intensity and encourage your nerves to follow suit.

3. J. S. Bach, "Air" from *Suite for Orchestra No. 3* (*Adagio Karajan Vol. 1*). A Baroque adagio clocking in at a stately fifty beats per minute, Bach's classic Air fills in the tempo gap from the previous number with a rich orchestral texture. The walking bass and warm harmonies gently coax you down, down, down . . .   *(continued . . .)*

4. El McMeen, "Fanny Power" (*Celtic Treasure*). Moving at forty-two beats per minute (counting each three-part pulse as a beat), this solo guitar piece is slower and much simpler than the Bach air, but a good deal of melodic movement keeps the drop in stimulus level from being too abrupt.

5. The Benedictine Monks of Santo Domingo de Silo, "Os iusti" (*Chant*). Voices float in unison, unaccompanied and unmetered, their long modal melodies echoing and mysterious. You float with them, no longer needing harmony or beat, freed from the structures of time and space that define your busy days.

No matter how overamped you are to begin with, vectored listening like this can help you achieve the tranquility of monks in the cloister in under twenty-five minutes.

Mind-Body Listening

Focused listening provides the deepest relaxation. When you have the leisure to devote yourself to total listening, try these imaging techniques to bring the tranquilizing power of music from your brain into your body:

• Lie on your back with your legs slightly apart and your arms at your sides with palms facing up (the yoga *savasana* relaxation pose). Think of your body as a sponge, absorbing the music through every pore. Breathe deeply in time to the music, letting the beat help regulate and deepen each inhalation and exhalation.

• Close your eyes to shut out visual distractions and feel the music pulsing gently against your muscles and nerves, relaxing them with every beat or tone.

• Focus on the third eye—defined in yoga practice as the spot in the middle of your forehead—and feel the sound resonate there.

• Visualize the music as an ocean. You're floating there, letting the waves of the music massage your muscles. Feel your weightlessness in the total support of the musical sea.

• Listen to the melody line and focus only on that. Let nothing enter your mind except for that tune—where it's been, where it is, where it's going. Let the melody pick up any distracting thoughts (I can't pay my taxes, I left the baby on the bus) and gently move them along.

- If you like you can add verbal instructions to cognitively reinforce music's physiological and psychological effects, and so enhance your relaxation response.[10] Mentally talk yourself through the process of relaxing one part of your body at a time, or make your own spoken-word tape and play it on a small cassette player while listening to music on the stereo.

An Ear Massage

You don't need a masseuse to get the relaxing benefits of body work. Try this ear massage the next time you need a rubdown:

- Put on some Relaxing music and lie down in a comfortable position.

- Picture the electrical impulses created by the sound waves as tiny massaging points, entering through your ears and flooding your head with relaxing warmth. Feel your brow soften and your jaw relax as you begin to breathe in time to the music.

- With each deep breath, feel the sound hum and purr through your neck, shoulders, arms, and all thirty-three vertebrae on your spine.

- Breathe the music deep into your stomach and lower back. Feel it touch your pubic bone, then spread like soft light down your legs and into your thighs, knees, calves, and ankles.

- Direct the relaxing pulse to the soles of your feet, and let it vibrate back up through your body.

- Finally, leave your body behind and listen to the music with your whole head, as if the sound were flooding straight into your mind. Surrender to the pulse and the tone and let the music make you breathe.

The Heartbeat Effect

When you're looking for comfort, music with the heartbeat effect can be like a return to the womb. Any Relaxing selection that moves at about eighty beats per minute should give you that just-right feeling. You can even take your own pulse first and choose the speed that synchs exactly with yours.

You can also use music *slower* than eighty beats per minute to help you *escape* your inner clock and spend some time outside the relentless pace of your daily rhythms. This is recommended for deep relaxation or sleep.

Chronic or On-Task Stress

If you're prone to chronic tension or you work in a stressful situation—like performing surgery—listen to Relaxing music throughout the day or task to act as an ongoing rein on your nervous system. Supplement your stress-busting soundtrack with a few breaks to free yourself of the feelings that can accumulate under stress (see chapter 6, Cleanse, if you're mad, or chapter 5, Uplift, if you're depressed).

Transient Stress

If, however, stress is an isolated event in your life, cropping up occasionally when your boss yells at you, your boyfriend doesn't come home, or before a speech, test, or performance, total relaxation is the most efficient antidote. Use the Mind-Body Listening techniques on page 62 for a focused relaxation session.

Stage Fright

Personal appearances like speeches, presentations, performances, and interviews can be measurably stressful, often raising your heart rate and flooding your bloodstream with the stress hormone cortisol and brain chemicals epinephrine and norepinephrine.[11] These reactions are designed to prepare you for peak performance, but they can also give you a case of counterproductive jitters. Shaking hands and heavy breathing rarely impress your audience.

If personal appearances give you stage fright, try five minutes with headphones and Relaxing music before the big moment. Close your eyes and focus on your breathing. Internalize the musical message of calm control, and take it with you when you go on.

Stress Breaks

When you want a quick way to clear your head of worries, take a walk in the fresh air with some Relaxing music on your Discman. The action will distract you while the music relaxes you.

Hear Your Way to Better Hemodynamics

Blood pressure problems? Don't substitute music for medical care, but do take advantage of the fact that Relaxing music has been proven to be effective in reducing both diastolic and systolic blood pressure. It's also been shown to reduce stress hormones in hypertensive patients.[12] For natural blood pressure control, schedule Relaxing listening sessions into the most stressful times of your day.

Stay Smooth

Be sure to stick with Relaxing music when you're feeling anxious. Stimulating music has been shown to aggravate anxiety even more than Relaxing music relieves it.[13]

Patience

As we approach the new millennium, every day seems to bring an increased need to wait—on the freeway, while a massive graphics file downloads from the Web, or as the board decides who to fire in the latest round of downsizing. We just weren't genetically programmed to have the patience that modern life requires. But music can help prolong your tolerance of the waiting game.

Carolyn, a salesperson who calls on clients all over the Boston area, is allergic to traffic. She also has zero tolerance for the top-forty music that dominates the radio, and has been known to cut people off with vicious intent when she hits the wrong button on the dial.

Carolyn's solution is cool jazz tapes, which save her from the pitiless chatter of radio DJs, keep her calm, and give her something interesting to focus on while she waits for her lane to start moving again. Now, with Miles Davis accompanying each turn of the odometer, Carolyn arrives at her meetings smiling and composed.

Sandy has a different type of patience problem. A busy mother and part-time paralegal, she'd become so accustomed to moving at hyperspeed that she couldn't slow the pace when she sat down to eat. Her power swallowing habits had put ten pounds on her body and given Sandy a permanent case of heartburn.

One night while out to dinner with her family, Sandy was enjoying the music of the restaurant's classical guitar player. As the waiter cleared the plates, she realized she'd only eaten half her dinner in the time it had taken everyone else to finish theirs—and she was perfectly satisfied. She gave the waiter her half-full plate and went home in complete digestive calm. Now Sandy starts every meal with an appetizer of acoustic strings and eats at a comfortable, healthy pace.

Marie is a mom in search of patience. "When I want to block out the kids, I listen to opera. It gives me something to focus on other than fighting children, which lets me remove myself and keep from losing my temper too much. And since I don't drive, it's the only way I can find space for myself."

One study found that music alleviated stress during a ten-minute wait among strangers;[14] another found it to cut down perceived waiting time in line at the bank.[15] In an experiment conducted in Japan, music that induced alpha brain waves caused subjects to underestimate the passage of time.[16] But the best evidence for music's time-compressing benefits comes from your own experience as a music listener. Intuitively, we all tend to turn to music to alleviate the frustrating effects of our harried lifestyles. Relaxing music can put you in a more patient mood, so use it whenever your fuse feels shorter than the task ahead.

Braintuning Basics: Patience

Plan on Patience

Many long waits, such as being stuck in traffic and long lines at the post office, are predictable, so come prepared:

- Plan on using your car stereo and some well-selected discs or tapes whenever you have to drive in traffic. A recent survey showed that over 40 percent of drivers in Los Angeles, which has been officially judged to have the worst traffic in the country, relax to music on the road.[17] Take a tip from the experts.

- Have your Discman on hand to wait in line at the bank, grocery store, post office, library, DMV, or ticket counter.

- Listen while you wait for a bus, train, or plane; for an appointment with your overbooked doctor, lawyer, or boss; for your computer to stop making that chewing noise and return to active status; or for your date.

Take Control

Does the canned music in the dentist's waiting room make you want to turn the drill on those responsible? Part of the pain of waiting is having to relinquish control over your own time and environment. Music of your own choosing—not necessarily what's playing on the office sound system or car radio—can return control to you. Think of your Walkman as an aural patience pill.

Speed Eating

Have you ever powered down a meal and eaten more than you needed because you were swallowing faster than your satiety signals could fire? Relaxing music can help slow the pace of your meals and make a more pleasant dining atmosphere.

If speed eating is overfeeding you, try this:

- Put on some Relaxing music *before* you serve the meal.

- Once the task of cooking or working or whatever you've been doing is finished, sit down and focus on the music for a minute or two.

- Serve and eat your meal, pausing between bites to listen. You'll probably eat less, enjoy it more, and tune into feeling full at just the right time.

People

The ancient Greeks used music to calm the behavior of belligerent drunks. You can also try it with your landlord, lawyer, or mechanic; when you're breaking up or firing someone; or at the family dinner table. In any difficult interpersonal situation, Relaxing music can quiet your nerves and free the flow of conversation. Studies from the United States to Shanghai show that listening to music promotes interaction and a sense of communal well-being among people, and that conversations are rated as more satisfying when music is playing in the background.[18]

Music also makes people more likely to say what they feel.[19] Even among groups of inmates in a psychiatric prison, listening to music led to significant relaxation, better moods, and happier thoughts,[20] so surely it can ease your encounter with the IRS agent.

By the same token, music can add a sense of relaxed bonhomie when you just want to enjoy time with your friends or family. Whenever easygoing interaction is your goal, Relaxing music can break down barriers and create a shared social space through sound waves. It can also help you *control* social situations, to keep everyone feeling friendly and satisfied with the exchange.

Nadia is a young professor who hosts a monthly dinner party where her friends gather to eat and drink long into the night. One such dinner found her facing an impending publication deadline and preparation for a new class, and she felt too overworked to turn an evening's engagement into a twelve-hour rage. But kicking people out was not Nadia's style. She needed a subtler strategy to put a pleasant, timely end to her party.

At eleven o'clock, Nadia changed the music from sixties soul—there had just been several loud group renditions of "Try a Little Tenderness"—to a mix of acoustic string music. As if on cue, everyone switched from wine to water, quieted their raucous singing to intimate conversation, and by midnight the guests were dreamily floating toward the door and thanking Nadia for a great time. She congratulated herself on a good party and the promise of a hangover-free morning.

Leslie faced a different kind of interpersonal dilemma. After twenty years of marriage, her father had just announced that he was divorcing her mother and leaving his job as comptroller of a manufacturing company to begin his own charter sailing endeavor. The announcement shocked and upset Leslie, and though she rarely had intimate conversations with her dad, she realized she needed to talk about this with him.

Leslie prepared for her one-on-one by programming a selection of slow symphonic movements onto her CD player, and found that the music, which she knew her dad liked, made her first words come out more easily— and her father's too. By the end of their talk, Leslie's father had revealed some of his hidden hopes and dreams and she was ready to work on understanding his decision with a different perspective.

Whether you're calming belligerent drunks or delving into intimate issues, Relaxing music can strengthen your connection to other people.

Braintuning Basics: People

Difficult Discussions

Though many people know from experience that music can enhance social interactions, few think to draw on this resource outside of parties. Music can be a good friend when you're dealing with a sticky relationship issue. Use it as an ally when you're quitting a job or firing someone. Let music facilitate your next deal, apartment lease, or argument with your insurance company. And don't even think of speaking to your mother without it.

- Play background music as you talk face-to-face, so you both (or all) can share the relaxing benefit.

- If you're on the phone, listen to music on your end. It's not as friendly as listening together, but it *is* a competitive advantage.

- If you must talk on someone else's turf and arriving with a boom-box just wouldn't be appropriate—in traffic court, for instance—listen to music directly beforehand and let it play back in your head as you start to speak.

Songs in the Key of People

Evidence suggests that music in a major key might be better than a minor key for freeing the flow of talk, and that Relaxing sounds encourage more sociable behaviors than hard rock and rap,[21] so save the big beats and sad harmonies for another time.

Chilling

For more festive interactions, remember:

- Relaxing music can encourage constructive social behaviors while it makes you feel good in each other's company.

- Gearing down the music toward the end of a party can help slow your guests' social pace and make them start to look forward to seeing their pillow.

Panic

Perhaps you've been gripped by one out of thin air. The dizziness, faintness, pounding heart, and shallow breathing known as panic attacks plague as many as one in seventy-five Americans. Panic attacks are all the more disturbing to their victims because nobody really knows what causes them or how to cure them. Although thought to have biochemical origins, panic can quickly become associated with external phenomena present at the moment, like crowds, cars, or tall buildings, and once the association is made, the phenomenon alone can trigger another attack.[22]

Some people find that music can interrupt the trigger-reaction cycle of panic attacks—and perhaps let you do things you thought you couldn't. Ramona, for instance, decided to take up driving four years after she'd stopped because of frequent panic attacks in the car. She armed herself with tapes of vocal music and hit Play whenever a tough merge, traffic jam, or past association started to make her dizzy. Just knowing she had music on her side helped Ramona succeed behind the wheel.

Relaxing music can defuse the threat posed by potential panic stimuli.[23] By providing autonomic nerve control to help keep your pulse and breathing in check, and filling your mind to prevent you from focusing on the cues that push your panic button, music might circumvent or lessen your personal panic response.

Braintuning Basics: Panic

Un-Press The Panic Button

Let music help you break the panic connection with these interventions:

- Make a tape of proven Relaxing music for trigger situations, whether driving in the car, riding in elevators, or giving speeches.

- For unexpected triggers, keep a Walkman cued up to Relaxing music on hand at all times.

- You might even be able to stay calm in a panic situation by *imagining* soothing music[24]—a useful tactic if you're not forearmed with a Walkman. Listen to a relaxing selection several times at home so that you can replay it in your mind, then try calling it up from memory the next time the world starts to spin.

Drugs or Ambient Dub?

Many people treat chronic anxiety and/or panic with prescription tranquilizers that work on your brain chemistry to inhibit the action of your autonomic nervous system. Benzodiazepines, for instance, stimulate gamma-aminobutyric acid, which sends slowdown signals to your pounding heart and panting lungs.

You should certainly work with your doctor to find the anxiety treatment that works best for you, but remember that music, too, has neurophysiological power—and it's cheap, all-natural, and fun.

Balance

The outer world we inhabit seems more complex and challenging every day. It's easy to settle for just getting to where we need to be, doing what we should, talking to the right people, and tackling the latest problems.

But you have an inner world, too, and most people would agree that it has needs. Whether you call it spirit, soul, essence, chi, psyche, center, or prana, your inner energy requires nourishment and care. A key to leading a more relaxed life lies in the restoration of balance between the exoteric, or outer world we live in on a daily basis, and the esoteric, or inner life.

Daniel works as a journalist and spends his time pursuing sources, flattering editors, and letting other people talk. "By the end of the day I've made nice to so many people that I've completely lost my sense of self. I'm harried and flustered—so I take twenty minutes with just me and my music to remember what I'm about before going out for the evening."

The need for balance can also run in the opposite direction. Tachana works at home alone as a technical writer. After a day alone in the intensely logical world of words, Tachana rebalances by going to a funk aerobics class at her health club and losing herself in the sound of the drums. "The music pulls me out of my head. I stop thinking about microchips and feel myself connect with other, bigger energies."

When you live too much in the world, listening to music can be a counterbalancing, inward-directed experience. It pulls you from the external environment into your own sonic space, filtering out the noises and distractions that inevitably try to pull you back to the world—a passing car, the cat's meow, your mate moving around somewhere else in the house. It activates areas on the right side of your brain, stimulating imagery and providing relief from the logical constrictions of daily life. And by providing an internal point of focus, music can free your consciousness from external concerns and help you relax at a deep, inner level.

But music also harmonizes you with the outer world through vibration—the subtle and constant movement of life. The round tones of a saxophone come from a vibrating reed. To play the flute, you vibrate an entire column of air. And to pluck or bow a string is to set a vibration in motion. You'll remember from science class that the atoms that make up matter never stop moving, so essentially the entire universe is vibrating like the reed, air, or string that make musical sound.

The theory of harmonics links music to all human and plant life via the mathematical proportions of consonant intervals, or the way tones vibrate with each other.[25] A related idea is sacred geometry, which describes and connects the musical frequencies of vitamins, minerals, amino acids, hormones, and gases. These theories draw on a mix of music and physics to express and explain the nature of the universe.

If you allow yourself to consider vibration as a metaphor for divinity or its essence, then music is its audible manifestation. Resonance can rebalance your inner self with the abundance of energy that surrounds you.

Braintuning Basics: Balance

Harmonic Listening

Let the idea of harmonics guide your musical meditation:

- Imagine the physical world vibrating with the music you hear. Maybe the flute resonates with rocks and earth, the guitar with the ocean, and that particular chord at the end of the phrase with the cells of your body.

- Now, expand the resonance out beyond the physical earth. Send the music into space and let it ring with the planets and the sun.

- Continue outward, stopping to feel each sympathetic vibration. Keep going farther and farther and see what you find.

Take an Inner Vacation

Many people have perfected the art of pampering their outer selves to stay sane in our high-stress world. Jacuzzis, massage, and trips to Cancún take care of part of you. But are you giving your inner self a chance to recreate, too?

A meditative session with music can be like Club Med for the spirit. Perhaps your vacation involves letting your soul sprawl out and bask in the warmth of an East African *mbira* ostinato. Or maybe you have a more adventuresome spirit that likes to take a hang glide on an Indian *santur* riff. Or your inner energy might prefer to recharge with a spa treatment of pure, unaccompanied vocals. See the discography for more about all the places music can take you for an inner vacation.

Meditation

Many forms of meditation can be used for relaxation as well as transcendence. By encouraging you to let go of conscious thought, meditation can help you shed the day's stresses and distractions. From the quiet relinquishing of yoga to the submission and literal vacation of possession trance, stopping your usual flow of thoughts can be both excellent discipline and a much-needed break for your busy mind. And music can be a powerful tool in attaining a meditative state.

In addition to stimulating the alpha brain waves conducive to meditation, music can literally occupy your cortex while you move to other planes.

There's no room to think of your mortgage or international politics when you're occupied by the sound of Gregorian chant, *shakuhachi* flute, or deep *didgeridoo* (Australian drone).

"I wouldn't even say I meditate," says Carlos, a physics professor. "But I do like to blank out my mind with music to give myself a break. I use headphones, put on something mesmerizing, forget about the nature of matter, and just bliss." As someone who makes his living with intense mind work, Carlos is pulling an instinctive balancing act.

When the pressures of living in an ever-expanding universe are weighing heavily on your mind, take a break with an unthinking musical meditation.

Braintuning Basics: Meditate

Clear Light

- Let music be light inside of you. As the sound passes through your inner ear, picture it as pure, clear, and electric, illuminating your head from within.

- First the music floods your mind, then washes over each vertebrae in your spine and radiates outward to every last finger and toe.

- Knowing that music continues to feed the light with every sound that hits your cochlea, sit back, relax, and glow like a lightbulb screwed into a socket.

Dark Night

Use Relaxing music to escape the natural and artificial light that burns into your eyes and mind during every conscious moment:

- Close your eyes and make the music a thick, dark, soft blanket that blocks out every beam of light.

- Feel the sound surround you completely like a cloak. It's like wearing a weightless sleep mask over your entire body.

Get Possessed

Trance might be the most complete abdication of conscious thought in human experience (without pharmacological help). It's normally done in the company of others, in the context of a complex ritual, but with music's help, you may find you can achieve trance at home.

- Choose some trance music from the discography at the end of the chapter. It should have a steady pulse and mesmerizing effect.

- Take some time to get into the groove. Listen for the voice in the music—an instrument, beat, or repeated phrase—and hear it knocking at your body's door.

- Let it knock for awhile, as long as it takes for you to feel ready. Now, slowly open yourself up to the music, like a door opening gradually and letting in first a shaft of light, then a wedge.

- Now the music illuminates, then floods your being with a blinding light. The door is wide open. Let it in.

The Zen of Repetitive Tasks

Zen philosophy suggests that you can find the object of meditation in daily life—and what better place than a tedious chore? Thoughtful minds can easily become frustrated with the repetitive nature of jobs like paying bills, chopping vegetables, filing, or cleaning the house, but happily, this can also be an opportunity for meditation and relaxation. Adding music to monotonous work can improve productivity, reduce errors, prolong your attention span, quicken your pace, and offer a real-life place for contemplation.

Try trance music for your next repetitive task, and let the most ordinary undertakings put you into an altered state.

Designer Meditation Music

Many contemporary composers promote their music as creating certain brain waves or synchronizing the hemispheres of the brain. While the brain's electrical activity is too complex to achieve simple synchronization, it's true that music can affect the speed of your brain waves,[26] strengthen electrical relationships between different areas of the brain,[27] and bridge the creative and analytical functions of the left and right hemispheres.[28] But the clinical research supporting these effects refers to a wide variety of real-life musical sounds and styles. You needn't limit your musical horizons to designer synthesizer sounds in order to expand your mind.

Sleep

One in ten Americans suffers from regular insomnia. Up to a third of the entire population has an occasional bout. And an estimated one million people in the United States get inadequate sleep.

The problem only gets worse as you age. About 80 percent of Americans experience disrupted sleep patterns by age fifty. Sweet dreams are even more elusive to aging women—the loss of estrogen associated with menopause can keep your eyes wide open long after the lights go out.

With sleeplessness a nationwide epidemic and Halcion out of favor, it's time to remember that music is a natural soporific.

The High Price of Sleep Loss

Children and young adults need almost ten hours of sleep a night. Some anthropologists believe that the eight hours of nightly darkness at the equator have programmed our sleep needs and circadian rhythms since the dawn of mankind. And yet, the average American's nightly dose of z's has dropped from eight to seven hours per night since the 1950s. What does this increased consciousness cost?[31]

- Neuron overuse and subsequent imbalances in the nervous system

- Decreased concentration, memory, and ability to cope with stress; increased reaction time

- Impaired immune system functioning

- A tendency to eat more

Brian is a healthy young guy who broke up with his girlfriend and took on two new sales accounts all in one week. The combination of an empty bed and a full mind made it hard to fall asleep for the first time in Brian's life. He tried self-medicating with Scotch, which worked until he found himself waking up several times during the night in the erratic patterns of alcohol-induced sleep, and facing most mornings with a mild hangover. He worried that his work performance was slipping just when he needed to prove himself.

One evening, Brian happened to flip on a classical music station while reading his latest demographic report. Bach's Goldberg Variations spun out in endless phrases, the stately pace of the piano slowing his pulse and brain waves, the steady volume soothing his frazzled nerves. The next thing Brian knew, he was horizontal and listening to white noise with half a good night's sleep behind him.

You probably experienced the music-sleep connection early in your life when your mother sang lullabies, which centuries of experience and recent clinical trials show to be the most effective way to soothe babies to sleep.[29] At the other end of the age spectrum, music has been found to be an effective sleep aid for the elderly, who are often plagued by chronic wakefulness.[30] Whether you're a confirmed insomniac or just wide-eyed once in awhile, music can help you sink into a delta-wave state.

To save yourself from the toll of sleep loss, try music as a natural way to nod off for better health and performance.

Braintuning Basics: Sleep

The Sleep Cycle

Falling asleep almost sounds like an accident, but the process entails biological cues thought to begin when the hormone melatonin and the neurotransmitter serotonin send sleepy signals to the body. Further nudges come from the reticular activating system and the cortex. Then,

- Blood pressure drops.

- Pulse rate decreases.

- Muscles relax.

- Basal metabolic rate drops by 10 to 30 percent, but gastrointestinal activity can increase (as you digest your dinner).

Relaxing music slows down all the vital signs associated with sleep. So feed your cortex some soothing sounds and head for REM.

Sound Sleep

Some people report that they can't go to sleep to music, but many of them are cueing up sounds that wake up their mind and body just as they're trying to shut them down. Here are some sound sleep principles:

- Pick something that *pleases* you, but nothing that particularly *interests* you, or gets you to thinking about that time when . . .

- Model the gradual slowdown that leads to sleep with the iso principle of musical mood induction. This method engages you at your waking energy level, then gradually unwinds toward unconsciousness. Make a tape that starts at a tempo and intensity that match the way you feel at bedtime, then gets slightly slower and lower in pitch with each selection. End with something very soft and slow, no more than sixty beats per minute, to decelerate your heart rate to the rhythm of sleep.

- Try using the same music to fall asleep to every night to create a conditioned response. Don't listen to this music while operating heavy equipment!—and change your sleep tunes after any bouts with insomnia.

- Use a bedside tape player or remote control so you can adjust the volume and, if you prefer, turn off the music just before you go to sleep.

- Vigorous daytime activity increases your chances of peaceful night-time slumber, so be sure to get moving to some Energizing music during the course of your day.

The Relax Music-Mood Checklist

❑ Slow tempo (eighty beats per minute or less; sixty to seventy-two beats per minute for full relaxation)

❑ Even, easy pulse

❑ Regular, smooth, flowing rhythms

❑ Continuous sound, without stops or interruption; reverberation

❑ Slow, sustained, stepwise melodies

❑ Repetition

❑ Soft to moderate, constant volume (sixty-five decibels or less)

❑ Low pitch

❑ Warm tone colors (acoustic strings, winds, organ)

❑ Simple, consistent texture

❑ Harmonic consonance

❑ Minor keys for a meditative feel; major for comfort and interpersonal concerns

Avoid high-pitched or piercing sounds, big beats, sudden changes, soaring melodies, and dissonance.[32]

Test Your Relaxation Response

Cooling out during a harried workday can be very different than going to sleep at night. Research shows that the relaxation effect of different types of music can vary with people and settings,[33] so the best thing to do is test your relaxation response in all the different situations in which you wish to calm down—to find out, for instance, that what works in bed may not be what's best for blissing out at the beach.

See page 24 in the introduction for instructions on testing your music-mood response. A Relax discography follows the quiz. Start by testing your favorite styles from the list and recording your results in the journal that follows.

The Relax Music-Mood Test

I Feel	Before Listening	After Listening	Change, Before to After
	(1–5)	(1–5)	(+ or –, 0–4)
Calm	_____	_____	_____
Loose	_____	_____	_____
Breathing easily	_____	_____	_____
Quiet	_____	_____	_____
Unwound	_____	_____	_____
Tranquil	_____	_____	_____
Soft	_____	_____	_____
Composed	_____	_____	_____
Mellow	_____	_____	_____
Serene	_____	_____	_____

Total Change:
Your Relaxation Response (0–40) _____

The Relax Music-Mood Journal

Date	Situation	Selection	Score
_____	_____	_____	_____
_____	_____	_____	_____
_____	_____	_____	_____
_____	_____	_____	_____
_____	_____	_____	_____
_____	_____	_____	_____
_____	_____	_____	_____
_____	_____	_____	_____
_____	_____	_____	_____
_____	_____	_____	_____
_____	_____	_____	_____
_____	_____	_____	_____
_____	_____	_____	_____
_____	_____	_____	_____
_____	_____	_____	_____
_____	_____	_____	_____
_____	_____	_____	_____
_____	_____	_____	_____
_____	_____	_____	_____
_____	_____	_____	_____

Braintuning Music: Relax

Vocals

The **human voice** made the first music and carries primeval emotional power. People can recognize the archetypal sound of **lullabies** even in other languages and musical styles[38]—suggesting a cross-cultural affinity to the sound of the female voice singing simple songs. It's like audio comfort food no matter what your age or ethnic identity.

A more sophisticated permutation is **early vocal music of the Western art tradition**. From Gregorian chant to the floating feel of Renaissance polyphony, the pure tone quality and long reverberation used in vocal music from previous ages can soothe your inner child or your grown-up, stressed-out self. Try it for meditation. Spiritual author Thomas Moore recommends meditating on the "melisma"—long, twisting melodies sung over one syllable—in Gregorian chant.

Then there's the all-purpose **song**. For relaxing purposes, songs that feature a solo singer and soft accompaniment are as effective as they are global and timeless.

Classical

If you've ever listened to a thunderous Wagner aria or the climax of a Beethoven symphony, you know that not all Western concert music is soothing—but some of it is. From the Baroque era all the way to contemporary times, the second movements of symphonies, sonatas, and concertos tend to be slow, often marked with the tempo indicator **adagio**, which means "at ease." Slow movements can add to your own ease; make a tape of your favorite ones or program them on your CD player.

You can also choose relaxing classical music from a chronological perspective. Most concert music was more stately and restrained before the Classical age, which began about the mid-18th century (from Haydn forward). Think **early—medieval, Renaissance, and Baroque**—when you want repose.

Or skip ahead a century. Many **Romantic** (c. 1800–1900) composers returned to a dreamy feel after the sprightly energy of the Classical era. This was the age of the nocturne, designed for sensitive spirits who needed a good reverie in order to recover from too much passion.

The Case for Real Music

Why bother with music? The past few decades have brought a boom in the marketing of Relaxation sounds that have little or nothing to do with music—ocean waves, whale sounds, synthesized tone pulses, subliminal suggestion, and a category of music composed specifically for relaxation without any other aesthetic benefits. A composer in the latter genre proudly trumpets his "uniquely new kind of music that contains no recognizable melody, rhythm or harmony."[34]

But a study that measured how different kinds of music influenced phone caller's patience while on hold found that so-called "relaxation" music resulted in the most hang-ups, while the least hang-ups came from callers treated to a tape of real music by jazz masters such as Miles Davis.[35] Furthermore, a comparison of people's response to classical music versus comparable "simulated music" reported subjects feeling "pleasantly relaxed or comfortable" to real music, but "unpleasantly weary" to the simulated stuff.[36] And studies of subliminal suggestion tapes conclude that auditory subliminals are not perceived, nor do they influence behavior or unconscious verbal or visual imagery.[37] All evidence suggests that if you love music, you'll find your truest relaxation response in the real thing.

Acoustic Strings & Winds

A plucked string or blown flute vibrates with a wordless peace. Acoustic instrumentals featuring the soft tone colors shown to evoke relaxation can be very calming; the discography samples selections from around the world.

Classic & Cool Jazz

The tinkle of piano like ice in a glass, the thick caress of the saxophone, the resonance of the acoustic bass deep in your solar plexus—small-band jazz can smooth out all your rough edges. The "cool" style that developed in the 1950s, featuring a laid-back tempo and performance style, is a musical chill pill.

Add the smooth sounds of Brazil to cool jazz, mix in a pinch of European Romanticism, and you get the intimate sound of **bossa nova**. Loaded with imagery of sun-drenched beaches, bossa nova can turn your bones to a very pleasant jelly.

When you want to relax, be careful not to confuse these styles with the upbeat sounds of bebop or the dissonance of avant-garde jazz.

Trance Music

Trance involves the idea of surrender—in this case, to music. In Haitian *vodou*, participants dance to drumming and singing until a climactic moment called *kase* in which the dancers are possessed by spirit guides or *Iwa* and lose contact with the conscious world. Similar music-trance connections are found in Brazilian *candomblé*, Sufi *dhikr*, Indonesian *gamelan*, East African Shona *mbira*, West African Yoruba ceremonies, and Moroccan Gnawa *derdebas*.

Things you can do in trance reportedly include walking on burning coals and piercing your flesh without bleeding. You can cure diseases, see into the future, speak in tongues, and chat with the dead. Or, you can just relax.

Ambient

Electronic musician Brian Eno pioneered "ambient" in the 1970s as a real-music version of Muzak, or background music. He said his richly-textured compositions were "intended to induce calm and a space to think," and his concept has proven popular enough in our society of stress to spawn **ambient dub**, which is like returning to the womb with a synthesizer under your arm.

The Braintuning Discography: Relax

STYLE	TITLE
Lullabies	• Pamela Ballingham. *A Treasury of Earth Mother Lullabies*. Earth Mother Productions 05B. Classics in a high, clear voice with simple, soothing accompaniment. • Beijing Angelic Choir. *Chinese Lullabies*. Wind Records 5013. A Chinese children's choir sings lullabies that translate as "Clear Moon, Quiet Winds," "Hammock Hanging between Betel Trees," and more. • *Billboard Family Lullaby Classics*. Hanna-Barbera Singers, Temple Kaye, Disney Studio Chorus, Rhino 72454. • *Celtic Lullaby*. Ellipsis Arts 4150. • Kids Praise. *Lullabies*. Word 3616. A children's a cappella vocal group.

• Listening to the World. *Lullabies and Children's Songs.*
Unesco 8102.
  • *Lullabies from Bohemia and Moravia.* Supraphon 111516.
  • Linda Ronstadt. *Dedicated to the One I Love.* Elektra 61916.
The pop star's favorite lullabies.

Gregorian Chant	• Hildegard von Bingen. *Canticles of Ecstasy.* Sequentia, Deutsche Harmonia Mundi 71850. This German abbess renowned as a mystic was one of the earliest known female composers in Western music.
	  • *Chant.* The Benedictine Monks of Santo Domingo de Silos, Angel 55138. The recording that broke chant in the modern world.
	  • *Salve Regina–Gregorian Chant.* Benedictine Monks of the Abbey of St. Maurice, Philips Silverline Classics 420879.

Early Vocal Music	• *An English Ladymass.* Anonymous Four, Harmonia Mundi 90780. Medieval chants and polyphony.
	  • Guillaume Dufay. *Music for St. Anthony of Padua.* Hyperion 66854.
	  • *The Emma Kirkby Collection.* Emma Kirkby, Hyperion 66227. Works by Bach, Handel, Dowland, Hildegard of Bingen, Machaut, and Monteverdi.
	  • Orlando de Lassus. *Lamentations of Jeremiah the Prophet.* Phillipe Herreweghe and La Chapelle Royale Vocal Ensemble, Harmonia Mundi 901299. An unchanging tempo, narrow range, and consonant harmonic scheme make these voices seem to float forever as they recount a book of the Old Testament. Pure and meditative.
	  • Guillaume de Machaut. *Messe de Notre Dame.* Andrew Parrott & the Taverner Consort, EMI Reflex 747949. One of the earliest polyphonic settings of the Mass Ordinary.
	  • *Music of the Gothic Era.* David Munrow & the Early Music Consort of London, Deutsche Grammophon 415292. Works by Machaut, Vitry, Perotin.
	  • Giovanni Pierliugi Palestrina. *Mass "Hodie Christus Natus Est" and Six Motets.* EMI Eminence 764045.
	  • *Vox Iberica I: Donnersöhne/Sons of Thunder.* Sequentia, Deutsche Harmonia Mundi 77199. Music from the 12th century codex at Santiago de Compostela.

Songs (folk, traditional, singer–songwriter, etc.)	• *African Voices: Songs of Life.* Narada 63930. Musicians from Kenya, Senegal, and Uganda perform traditonal and composed songs.
	  • Anita Baker. *Rapture.* Elektra 60444. Like pouring warm liquid into your head.
	  • *Celtic Spirit.* Narada 63929. Celtic songs in both folk and enriched arrangements.

- Tracy Chapman. *Tracy Chapman*. Elektra 60774.
- Cowboy Junkies. *Lay It Down*. Geffen 24952.
- Enya. *Watermark*. Reprise 26774. Irish vocalist blends Celtic and New Age styles.
- Emmylou Harris. *Wrecking Ball*. Elektra/Asylum 61854. A voice of purity with dreamlike arrangements.
- Carole King. *Tapestry*. Epic 34946. The singer-songwriter's 1971 classic.
- k.d. lang. *All You Can Eat*. Warner Brothers 46034. Cool jazz meets country and pop.
- Loreena McKennitt. *The Visit*. Warner Brothers 26880. Celtic folk.
- Sarah McLachlan. *Fumbling Toward Ecstasy*. Arista 18725.
- James "Bla" Pahinui. *Mana*. Dancing Cat 38033. Traditional and classic Hawaiian songs rendered with rich vocal vibrato and accompanied by slack key guitar.
- Shusha. *Persian Love Songs and Mystic Chants*. Lyrichord 7235. Cool Eastern vocals with flute and *zarb* drum.
- James Taylor. *Greatest Hits*. Warner Brothers 3113.
- *Troubadours of the Folk Era, Vol. 2*. Rhino 70263. Pete Seeger, Tim Hardin, and other well-known folkies.
- Neil Young. *Harvest*. Reprise 2277.
- Your favorite artist unplugged.

Symphonic Slow Movements

- *Adagio Karajan 1 and 2*. Herbert von Karajan and the Berlin Philharmonic, Deutsche Grammophon 445282 and 449515. Great classical slow movements from Vivaldi to Mahler.
- Ludwig van Beethoven. Second movement, *Symphony No. 6*. Leonard Bernstein & the Vienna Philharmonic, Deutsche Grammophon 413779. This pastoral movement is a good candidate for focused listening to take your mind off your worries.
- Henryk Górecki. Second movement of *Symphony No. 3* (*"Symphony of Sorrowful Songs"*). David Zinman & the London Sinfonietta, Elektra Nonesuch 79282. This heartbreakingly beautiful piece for soprano and orchestra seems to make time stand still.
- Wolfgang Amadeus Mozart. Second movement, *Symphony No. 40* on *Symphonies No. 35-41*. Carl Böhm & the Berlin Philharmonic, Deutsche Grammophon 447416. A delicate figure cascades through the orchestra; perfectly symmetrical phrases help you rebalance from the inside out.
- The second movement of your favorite symphony, sonata, or concerto.

Romantic Piano	• Johannes Brahms. *Intermezzi Op. 118 No. 2 and Op. 117 No. 1*. Ivo Pogorelich, Deutsche Grammophon 437460. Dreamy piano induces instant reverie. • Frederic Chopin. *Nocturnes*. Maria João Pires, Deutsche Grammophon 447096. 21 piano lullabies; let each one take you deeper. • Claude Debussy. *Beau Soir* on *Berlin Recital*. Anna-Sofie Mutter, Deutsche Grammophon 445826. Violin and piano paint the picture of this "beautiful night," ending with one perfect note. • Erik Satie. *Piano Music Vol. 1*. Virgin 59515. One of the first "serious" composers to write music especially to soothe the stressed-out modern man; liked to play late-night Paris honky-tonks.
Acoustic Strings & Winds	• J.S. Bach. *The Goldberg Variations*. Harmonia Mundi 7901240. Composed for a Russian count who complained of insomnia, these harpsichord variations unwind a theme in much the same way that you drift off to sleep. • Keola Beamer. *Mauna Kea—White Mountain Journal*. Dancing Cat 38011. If sound can resemble basking on a sunny beach, Hawaiian slack key guitar does so with strings loosened into easy open tunings. In the Hawaiian language there's a word for such relaxing songs: *nahenahe*. • Tarun Bhattacharya. *Kirvani*. Music of the World 139. An extended rag on the *santur*, or Indian hammered dulcimer, with *tabla* accompaniment. • *Fantasies, Ayres, and Dances*. The Julian Bream Consort, RCA Victor 7301. Elizabethan viols, lutes, and flutes. • Gour Goswami and Steve Gorn. *The Indian Bamboo Flute: Two Masters in Tradition*. Lyrichord 7387. One *rag* for twilight, another for late night, performed on the Indian *bansuri* flute. • *Guitar Works*. Narada 61032. Contemporary, mostly acoustic compositions performed on classical, steel string, 12-string, 10-string, scalloped fretboard, and harp guitars. • Ali Jihad Racy. *Ancient Egypt*. Lyrichord 7347. Composed to accompany the King Tut exhibit and inspired by the Egyptian Book of the Dead. Performed on Near Eastern instruments such as *nay* (flute), *buzuq* and *'ud* (lutes), and *mizmar* (oboe). • Tadashi Tajima. *Shingetsu*. Music of the World 124. Japanese *shakuhachi* flute. These *hokyoku*, original sacred pieces from Zen Buddhism, feature empty spaces and breath in a style called *suizen*, or "Blowing Zen."
Classic & Cool Jazz	• *Great Vocalists of Jazz—The Voice of the Soul*. Esquire/Blue Note 32994. Swank tunes by Nat King Cole, Billie Holiday, Chet

Baker and more, compiled by the experts of smooth at Esquire magazine.

• Chet Baker. *Let's Get Lost; The Best of Chet Baker Sings*. Pacific Jazz/Capitol 92932. Musicians on heroin often make relaxing music (with Charlie Parker and Kurt Cobain shining exceptions to the rule). These 1953–56 sessions capture the cool sound of the trumpeter and vocalist.

• *John Coltrane and Johnny Hartman*. GRP/Impulse 157. Hartman was a seminal crooner, and "Lush Life" the quintessential lounge song.

• The Miles Davis Quintet. *Relaxin' with the Miles Davis Quartet*. Prestige OJC-190. Miles's cool, muted trumpet blows ballads alongside John Coltrane, Red Garland, Paul Chambers, and Philly Joe Jones.

• The Bill Evans Trio. *The Artist's Choice: Highlights from "Turn Out the Stars: The Final Village Vanguard Recordings."* Warner Brothers 46425. The pianist's final recordings from New York's Village Vanguard.

• Billie Holiday. *Billie Holiday Sings Standards*. Verve 27650. Jimmy & Stacy Rowles. *Looking Back*. Delos 4009. Dad on piano and daughter on flügelhorn.

• George Shearing and Mel Torme. *An Elegant Evening*. Concord Jazz 4294. Lush piano and the vocal velvet fog.

• Zoot Sims. *For Lady Day*. Pablo 2310-942. Zoot wraps his deep, warm tenor sax around songs made classic by Billie Holiday.

• *Lester Young Trio*. Verve 521650. 1946 session with Nat King Cole and Buddy Rich by one of the most important tenor sax players in history.

Bossa Nova	• Astrud Gilberto. *Look at the Rainbow*. Verve 821556. • João Gilberto. *The Legendary João Gilberto*. World Pacific 793891. • *The Girl from Ipanema: The Antonio Carlos Jobim Songbook*. Verve 525472.
Trance Music	• The Erguner Brothers. *Preludes to Ceremonies of the Whirling Dervishes*. JVC World Sounds 5005. Ethereal Sufi flute, deep drums—and the dervishes prepare to whirl. • *Global Meditation: Authentic Music from Meditative Traditions of the World*. Ellipsis Arts 3210. The place to start if you want to sample the spirit and trance musics of the world. This 4-CD set has it all—Buddhist chant, *didgeridu*, *vodou*, *gamelan*, *qawwali*, and much more in high-quality, authentic recordings. The discs are sequenced for contrast and you might find the juxtaposition of styles impractical for meditation or trance (though it makes for beautiful

listening)—but you can compile your own meditation tapes from this wealth of material, or use the selections as jumping-off points for further exploration.

• Thomas Mapfumo & the Blacks Unlimited. *Chamunorwa (What Are We Fighting For?)*. Mango 539900. An electric guitar version of East African *mbira* music.

• Dumisani Maraire & Ephat Mujuru. *Shona Spirit*. Music of the World 136. Two of the greatest living *mbira* players from Zimbabwe unite in hypnotic, circular trance pieces.

• *Trance 1 and 2*. Ellipsis Arts 4000 and 4010. Compilations of authentic trance music with extended selections long enough to escape from the rhythms of this world. Disc 1 includes Sufi flute music of the whirling dervishes, Tibetan Buddhist chant, and Indian *dhrupad* (vocal music to *tanpura* drone accompaniment.) Disc 2 is Sufi chanting from Chinese Turkestan, hypnotic Moroccan Gnawa music, and Balinese *gamelan*.

Ambient	• Harold Budd. *Pavillion of Dreams*. EG/Carolina 30. Harps, marimbas, voices—Budd's work of "existential prettiness" marked his return after "minimalizing himself out of a career." • Brian Eno. *Ambient 1—Music for Airports*. EG/Caroline 17. Eno's music could bankrupt the pharmaceutical industry, but his less-skilled imitators have camouflaged the achievements of one of the few true mood musicians. • *Ambient 4—On Land*. EG/Caroline 20. Created to combat the stress of life in New York City, which requires a strong musical antidote. • Vicki Hansen. *Earth Heart*. Australian Music International 5005. Ambient keyboard layering over Australian *didgeridu* and other drone sounds. • *A Journey Into Ambient Groove: Messages from Within and Without*. Quango/Island 444072. Cool and delicious grooves of the European school. • The Orb. *U.f.orb*. Island 5006.
Delta Waves Sound	• Dr. Jeffrey Thompson. *Brainwave Suite: Delta*. Relaxation Company 3053. Sound pulses said to create delta brainwaves, the electrical frequencies of sleep. Accompanied by Tibetan bowls and nature sounds.
The Heartbeat Effect	• Randy Crafton. *Inner Rhythms*. Relaxation Company 3185. American composer uses world percussion and the iso principle of starting at a tempo he attributes to the heartbeat under stress, then gradually slowing down to 57 bpm in a trance-like piece for African *mbira*.

See page 255 for Sources.

Relax: The Braintuning 5

A diverse sampling from the discography to get you started:

- Orlando de Lassus. *Lamentations of Jeremiah the Prophet.* Phillipe Herreweghe and La Chapelle Royale Vocal Ensemble, Harmonia Mundi 901299.

- Keola Beamer. *Mauna Kea—White Mountain Journal.* Dancing Cat 38011.

- *Adagio Karajan 1 and 2.* Herbert von Karajan and the Berlin Philharmonic, Deutsche Grammophon 445282 and 449515.

- *Great Vocalists of Jazz—The Voice of the Soul.* Esquire/Blue Note 32994.

- Dumisani Maraire & Ephat Mujuru. *Shona Spirit.* Music of the World 136.

I Am the Most Serene

Now you know the audio antidote to stress and anxiety: Keep it low and slow. Whether you choose music that feels like a warm massage or a cool compress, use mind-body listening to apply soothing sounds directly to your jangled nerves. Let the music sweep unwanted thoughts from your mind and tension from your muscles.

Skip Relaxing music when you're depressed, before or during a vigorous workout, or when you need to maintain maximum alertness (driving, reading, or working). Otherwise, surrender—and be most serene.

Three

....

Focus

Neurological evidence proves that Mozart makes you smarter. But perhaps you didn't know that Pink Floyd can enhance your memory, or that Bizet can help you learn Hamlet, or even that the Lemonheads can teach you math. Music's power for learning and brainwork goes far beyond Mozart. Let it make you a mental giant.

Focus Overview

Focusing Music Can Help You With:	Use These Techniques if You Are:	How Music Helps:
Abstract Reasoning	Working with mathematical or scientific theory; undertaking spatial or visual tasks	Stimulates structured neural firing that primes your right brain for high-level thinking
Learning and Recall	Studying language, vocabulary, math, or facts	Induces receptive mood; encodes information in the mind

| Brainwork (analytical, creative, administrative, etc) | Seeking to work harder and faster. | Enhances concentration and attention span by alleviating task anxiety, boosting arousal levels, filtering out distracting noise, and providing structured movement through time. |
| Motivation | Unenthusiastic; mentally distant; sitting down to work session on a large-scale venture like a dissertation or prospectus. | Acts as Pavlovian cue; provides reward for progress. |

Though we tend to associate music with leisure time activities, it can also be a useful tool when you're trying to be bright and efficient. The Introduction described how neural networks are created in your cortex when you listen to music. Now you'll learn how to translate this process into a cognitive edge.

Music has the neural firepower to jazz up your math and reasoning skills. Listening to music while you learn material can help you encode information and improve its recall. During a long workday, you can use music to induce a mood of concentration, filter out distractions, and structure your thoughts. A project-specific soundtrack can set the tone for Herculean undertakings, keeping you on task while rewarding your progress along the way. Whether it's harmonizing the hemispheres of your brain or simply supporting you in a time of challenge, music can help you think and work harder and better.

Abstract Reasoning

Mozart Makes You Smarter (At Least for Ten Minutes in Higher Math)

You may have heard about the "Mozart makes you smarter" discovery by researchers at the University of California–Irvine Center for the Neurobiology of Learning and Memory in 1993. For this experiment, thirty-six college students prepared for an IQ test in three different ways. In one round, they sat in silence—the way many of us, conditioned by years of quiet classrooms and libraries, tend to prepare for high-level thinking—then underwent a grueling round of pattern analysis, multiple-choice matrices, and paper figure visualization tests. In another trial they listened to a spoken relaxation tape, which would seem like a good way to fight the stress of a test, then performed the same group of exercises. But the best test preparation turned out to be listening to ten minutes of Mozart's Sonata for Two Pianos in D Major, after which the students registered mean IQ scores *nine points higher* than when they had prepared in silence, and *eight points higher* than after the relaxation tape. These whiz kids could write home that college was going great; today, with a little musical help, their IQ had hit 119.[1]

The news was groundbreaking enough to make the national media: Ten minutes of music make a nine-point difference in IQ! Students, educators, and everyone with brainy ambitions rejoiced. Mozart was cheaper and more edifying than smart drinks—and now, scientifically proven.

The UC experimenters hypothesize that the cognitive jolt comes when music excites neurons and causes them to fire over large regions of the cortex in the same kinds of patterns used in abstract reasoning, and that the resulting neural networks prime your mind for high-level thinking. Specifically, the researchers propose that complex, highly structured, non-repetitive music like compositions of the Western classical era stimulates this sort of structured neural firing.

It's significant that the improved test scores were not related to an increase in pulse rate, supporting the experimenters' theory that the music was operating at the neural, not the nervous system level. In other words, this is not the extra-cup-of-coffee-you'll-regret-later kind of fix. This is music actually *hot-wiring your mind.*

Now, the caveats. First, the IQ enhancement in the experiment was temporary, lasting only for the ten to fifteen minutes required for the tests. That won't get you through the average midterm or discovering the next theory of relativity. Secondly, the boost is only proven for *spatial-temporal reasoning*, a right-brain function that helps you with higher math, science, chess, and certain other types of abstract thinking (Einstein's brain was found to have twice the normal amount of neuron-support cells in the spatial-reasoning area[2]), but not with verbal reasoning: reading, vocabulary, writing, and other such analytical tasks. And third, there's been no testing to determine which musical characteristics of the Mozart selection contributed to the IQ enhancement. All we know is that a second trial of the experiment using dance music and a composition by Philip Glass—much more repetitive than Mozart—failed to raise test scores, just as the researchers had predicted.

Alas, another Mozart experiment at North Carolina Wesleyan College by a research team using a different spatial reasoning test found no significant IQ boost from music.[3] But the UC team did succeed in duplicating the experiment and its results in a separate follow-up trial,[4] suggesting that the two IQ tests may have measured different types of spatial reasoning.

Evidence on the music-IQ link is still preliminary, but the notion that a few minutes with Mozart might excite the neurological networks you need for abstract reasoning could revolutionize the way we think about music.

The UC-Irvine experiment departed from the mainstream of research on music cognition by addressing the process of *listening to* rather than *performing* music. In fact, the team took an earlier discovery of a correlation between musical *performance* ability and spatial-visual skills,[5] and expanded their hypothesis into the realm of listening. The important news is that you don't need to play like Mozart to enjoy the cognitive benefits of music. Just listen—and let the virtuosity of those hardworking musicians rub off.

Music & Neural Priming: History in the Making

1985: Researchers find a correlation between music cognition and spatial reasoning. The discovery involves performing, not listening to music, and there is little immediate response from the world at large.[6]

1991: Xiaodan Leng and Gordon Shaw create a computer model of neural firing patterns in the cortex that generates music similar to Baroque and other compositional styles, suggesting that music mimics cortical activity.[7] Shaw joins with Frances Rauscher and other researchers at UC-Irvine and they fire up to find a causal relationship between musical processing and the ability to reason.

1993: The team proves their hypothesis: Ten minutes of a Mozart sonata improve scores on the spatial reasoning portion of an IQ test by eight to nine points. Furthermore, a pilot study concludes that ten three-year-olds score substantially better on a spatial reasoning test after receiving a few months of music lessons. The researchers postulate that musical activities help systematize neural firing patterns in the cortex to assist with other pattern development tasks. *(continued)*

1994: The team replicates its IQ findings with Mozart and expands the study with three-year-olds to include thirty-three subjects who receive weekly piano and daily singing lessons for eight months. The results: The toddlers taking music lessons score significantly better on spatial reasoning tasks than the control group.[8]

1997: The preschool study grows. Now involving seventy-eight children and including a group from an inner-city school, the study administers biweekly piano lessons and daily singing lessons to one test group and singing lessons alone to another. A third group receives computer keyboard lessons twice a week, and the control group gets no lessons at all. After six months, the children receiving piano and singing lessons score 34 percent higher on spatial reasoning tests than the other three groups, who show no improvement. Furthermore, the effect lasts at least one day, which suggests a long-term change. Conclusion: Studying piano assists in cognitive development, and the computer keyboard is no substitute.[9]

Further experiments about the connection between music and abstract reasoning are in the works, and there may have been more discoveries made by the time you read this. One thing is clear: These studies are making history, right now in the present. The question is what society, long accustomed to considering the arts an optional if decorative add-on to education and cognitive development, will do with this new information. Will you take some time to listen to complex music? Will you buy your three-year-old a piano? Are we ready to recognize music as an essential component of human intelligence?

Must It Be Mozart?

These newfound connections between music and the kind of reasoning that supports higher math should come as no surprise. All of Western music theory is based on an abstract construct by Greek mathematician Pythagorus that determines which notes go together, in scales, keys, and chords, by calculating the ratios between their frequencies and overtones. To discuss the rules underlying Western music, from classical to rock, folk, and jazz, is to embark upon a dizzying journey of numbers, fractions, and series for which you *need* some neural priming!

There's still a lot to learn about why Mozart's music in particular has an IQ-enhancing effect in this particular cognitive area, and what other sorts of music might trigger similar neurological responses. The working theory is that the benefit comes from Mozart's complexity: melodies are continually transformed, and new melodic and harmonic ideas introduced. If the perceptual process involved in following a melodically and harmonically complex composition activates cortical firing patterns used in other cognitive activites, then all this musical processing might translate into a sort of mental aerobics.

But were the college students in the experiment really following the music? Would Mozart have had the same neurological effect on, say, Indonesians or Indians, who have complex music traditions of their own? What if you were to repeat the experiment with a musical sample that was equally complex but less well-loved—like Stockhausen or Sun Ra? Until we know the answers to these questions, we can't give Mozart a corner on the cognitive market. Complex musics are found in cultures around the world, and it's possible that many different musical styles can stimulate the neural firing that elevates the spatial-temporal or other components of IQ.

An experiment testing the mood effect of different composers in the Western art tradition found Mozart to have neutral mood results (versus a depressive rating for Beethoven and a positive effect for Aaron Copland).[10] This correlates with the music's neutral effect on pulse rate in the Irvine experiment. Maybe it's the very mood neutrality of Mozart's music that allows it to operate at the cognitive level. If you subscribe to the Mr. Spock theory of logic, you can't expect to do your best abstract reasoning while having an emotional experience.

Braintuning Basics: Abstract Reasoning

Listening for High-Level Reason

Music can prime your mind for deducing math theorems, drawing conclusions from a chemistry experiment, playing chess, or any abstract thinking challenge. Are you grappling with parabolas, or the crazy lines created by calculus and differential equations, or all those 3-D graphs meant to depict financial performance these days? Try the following techniques with right-brain complex music from the discography at the end of the chapter:

- Listen *before* you undertake your task. You're aiming for a priming, or warm-up effect, and demanding background music might actually create a "dual task paradigm" and distract you.[11]

- Focus on the themes, or sentences of melody. Remember them, follow them, hear them change and pass from one instrument to the next.

- Feel the neurons firing in your head, creating elegant, logical, electrical maps, just like wiring a circuit board.

- Use interval listening to refresh your neural firing patterns—take a quick music break every fifteen minutes or so. Note that the exact timing of music's IQ-boosting effect is not yet thoroughly tested, so do whatever works for you.

For more on right-brain priming, see chapter 7, Create.

Listening for Language and Logic

It hasn't been clinically tested, but why not try music to prime the left brain, too? While the Mozart experiment hypothetically localized the music's cognitive benefits in the right brain, where melodic and harmonic information is processed, it seems to follow that music with complex rhythm, which is processed mostly in the left hemisphere, could prime your neural networks for the language and logic operations that also take place there. To take a leap into the possibilities of left-brain priming, which might help with reading, writing, and analytical tasks, choose some music from the left-brain selections in the discography and:

- Listen for ten minutes or so before you begin your cognitive task, then turn off the music. As with right-brain priming, you want to prepare for, not compete with, your thinking.

- Concentrate on sequential thought: Listen carefully to the rhythms. Try to identify how beats are grouped together in time, and how the patterns change from one group to the next. Compare what's happening now with what you just heard and try to predict what might come next.

- Clap or tap your toe along with the basic underlying pulse. With metrically complex music, this can be harder than it sounds.

- Sense the electricity in the left side of your head as your cortex encodes, analyzes, remembers, and predicts the sequences you hear.

- Refresh your analytical mind with additional listening breaks as needed.

Learning and Recall

Listen While You Learn

Mozart's kick to your spatial-temporal reasoning is great when you need to figure out an abstract problem, but what if you need to learn a language, or the capital cities of the world? Music is a proven learning aid, too, but in contrast with the reasoning boost given by complex music, it seems to be simpler sounds that drive lessons home, especially when it comes to the world of facts, words, and formulas.

James thought he had hit the wall in business school. He was failing a theoretical course on economic risk that involved more Greek symbols and formulas than his mind could manage. By the time he came across an ad for a music tape that promised to improve memory, he was ready to try anything.

James's roommate was a little worried when he came home to find James chanting Greek formulas to a Baroque concerto. But James, though doubtful, thought the facts just might be sinking in faster. Studying was certainly more pleasurable now, and maybe he was spending more time on the work than before.

The final proved it. Formulas flowed from his mind to his blue book in measured phrases, and his grade proved James a master assessor of economic risk. He wasn't sure if Morgan Stanley or Goldman Sachs would forgive him the F on the midterm, but he would certainly get points for his mid-period turnaround.

Theory on *why* music works as a learning aid has lagged behind wide-ranging evidence that it *does*, for math, language, reading, and memorizing facts. One possibility is that music induces a receptive mood that enhances cognitive processes in general. It might serve as a mnemonic memory aid to help you encode information in the mind. Whether you learn to background music or sing new words or concepts out loud, music seems to help initial learning, recall, and transference into working memory.[12]

In clinical studies, Pink Floyd's "The Wall" helped preteenage boys remember spoken numbers.[13] Memorizing multiplication tables to music improved retention for both normal and learning-disabled students.[14] Everyone who learned "Conjunction junction, what's your function?" with ABC's "Schoolhouse Rock" show has experienced music's memory-enhancing power firsthand. The 1970s series revived a nineteenth-century schoolroom practice of memorizing facts by singing them to popular tunes like "Yankee Doodle." The cast of the TV show *Gilligan's Island* taught TV audiences Shakespeare's *Hamlet* when they set it to familiar tunes from *Carmen*. If you've ever found yourself singing "Neither a borrower nor a lender be" to the tune of "March of the Toreadors," you were one of Gilligan's students.

Some music researchers have taken the idea of learning to music a step further. The "accelerated learning" school pioneered by Bulgarian psychologist Georgi Lozanov during the 1950s and '60s and popularized in the United States by Sheila Ostrander and Lynn Schroeder holds that learning in time to music moving at about sixty beats per minute helps imprint material in your memory with less conscious effort.[15] This technique— which assisted James through his economic risk exam—is considered best-suited for memory-based tasks like learning languages, definitions, facts, and formulas. Proponents of musically accelerated learning assert that it can help you learn five to ten times faster and recall the material with greater ease, and there are some experimental results to back this claim.[16]

Learning to music is certainly an improvement on the usual grind of silent memorization. Why shouldn't something that sounds good make your memory work better?

Reading

Music has also proven useful in acquiring verbal sequencing skills, or language. Whether in teaching language and reading basics to preschoolers or a second language to older students, music helps with learning, recall, and discrimination.[17] In Thailand, the public school system uses songs to practice tonal aspects of the language.[18] In the United States, matching melodies to sentences significantly increased accuracy in verbal inflection for English as a Second Language students, while in France, some educators advocate using pop music to teach the vocabulary, syntax, and cultural context of foreign languages to teenagers.[19]

There's some debate about music's net impact when it comes to reading comprehension. Some scholars believe that because so much music processing takes place in the right brain, it might compete for attention with language centers in the left.

But studies also suggest that the *proper* music can actually enhance reading comprehension. One experiment found that reading to classical music boosted comprehension, but rock music distracted readers.[20] Results from another trial showed that studying to familiar and preferred music raised comprehension scores.[21] And in an experiment with below-average readers, listening to rap music, composing rap songs, and discussing the lyrics' message increased reading proficiency for fifth- and sixth-graders.[22]

Furthermore, music can facilitate letter recognition, figural fluency, pictorial memory, and perhaps other spatial skills—probably by activating neurons in the right hemisphere. In one study, increasing the music's tempo actually increased reading speed.[23]

It does appear that unfamiliar or distracting music can interfere with reading comprehension, but the jury is still out on the specifics of music and reading. When a researcher measured the impact of background rap music on reading comprehension scores, the results varied by gender, listening habits, academic achievement, and personality. Evidence suggests that music might distract females from their reading more than males, so be sensitive to your own level of focus if you choose to read to music.[24]

Teach Your Children Well

Crosby, Stills, and Nash must have known that music was a good medium for teaching when they wrote their hit song. The new generation of superparents who discuss college options while the prospective student is still *in utero* will want to know about the jump start music can give young minds.

Early twentieth-century educators Carl Orff and Zoltán Kodály were pioneers in using music to help kids learn, proposing that it enhanced children's ability to concentrate and so supported better language development, reading ability, and coordination.[25] Their contemporary in Austria, Rudolf Steiner, integrated music into the curriculum of his Waldorf schools, which are currently going strong in the United States.[26] More recently, music educator and former elementary school teacher Don Campbell has proposed that music helps in the classroom by making connections in the brain and integrating experience into memory.[27]

But even more than a classroom tool, music at a young age might develop cognitive skills that have a long-term impact on the mind. Some scientists, including the UC-Irvine team, postulate that musical training at an early age, while the cortex is still "plastic," might cause *permanent* changes to the brain. In one study, musicians who started training before age seven had significantly larger corpus callosums (the corpus callosum bridges both sides of the brain and is important to interhemispheric communication) than others.[28] Another found that string players had larger cortical representations of the fingers of the left hand, and that the effect was greater, the younger the person had started to play.[29] Brain wave coherence, which reflects the number of functional interconnections in the brain, has been found to be greater both within and between hemispheres in people with musical training.[30]

A curriculum that used music to emphasize sequenced skill development from kindergarten through second grade significantly raised math scores in comparison with control groups for each grade—and the edge over the traditional curriculum increased as kids spent more time in the program.[31] And most dramatically, three separate experiments by the UC-Irvine team have concluded that giving three-year-olds piano and singing lessons raises their spatial and temporal reasoning test scores by as much as *80 percent.*[32]

It's been proposed that music works as a prelanguage that can be used to exercise the brain for higher cognitive functions.[33] Or maybe music is actually a postlanguage that plumbs our mental potential like no other process can.

Developing the Musical Mind

Children develop their music cognition during early years, while they might actually be organizing their cortexes for future mental efforts. Newborns to one-year-olds are drawn to rhythms, like Mom's heartbeat that they so recently left behind, and to rich, simple sounds. But babies less than six months old can sing back pitches sung to them,[34] and infants can recognize out-of-tune notes and changes in melodies as early as four months to a year.[35]

Preschoolers are enthusiastic explorers of music, which can pique their interest in other topics, too.[36] It's a good sign when children develop favorite songs—meaning they've activated the neural networks required to encode the tones, rhythms, and patterns involved, as well as the ability to compare them to a new event, judge them as the same, and say, "Mom! More Barney!" But neurological researchers might recommend that you play more Mozart and less Barney for the benefit of the cognitive processes that complex music seems to stimulate.

Braintuning Basics: Learning and Recall

Music for Memory

When studying for a test, embarking on long-term research, or preparing for a presentation, let music help you lock what you learn into memory with these tips for a background soundtrack:

- Choose familiar music, and keep it steady in tempo and dynamics so it doesn't distract you from your task.[37] If you find yourself stuck on a sentence while your spirit soars with a musical phrase, you've chosen wrong.

- If possible, listen to the same music to recall material as you did when you learned it. Psychological theory proposes that your memory becomes associated with the emotional context during which events took place, so recreating the mood with music can help access elusive facts.[38]

Accelerated Learning

To learn facts, formulas, or vocabulary, take your musical study session a step further with Ostrander and Schroeder's interpretation of Lozanov's accelerated learning techniques:[39]

- Put on some Baroque music that moves at about sixty beats per minute and features high strings like violin, guitar, mandolin, or harpsichord. The second movements of concertos by Bach, Telemann, or Vivaldi fill the bill—or see the discography.

- Listen to the music for a few minutes and try to breathe in time to the four-beat bars.

- When you feel relaxed and in tune with the tempo, have a partner read aloud the material you want to master, alternating data and silence with each four beats. Or make a tape of your material in advance, if you lack a learning partner.

- Continue for about twenty minutes, then finish by listening to a brief "allegro" section that moves at a brisk, lively pace to return to the workaday world.

Sing Yourself Smart

You can also commit things to memory—names and dates, addresses, theorems, Shakespeare passages, verb conjugations, legal documents, recipes, etc.—by singing along. To devise your own version of *Schoolhouse Rock* or *Hamlet* à la *Gilligan's Island*:

- Pick a recording without lyrics, containing one or more melodies you know well. Instrumental pop, classical marches and overtures, or anything else with a memorable tune and no words (at least on this recording) will do.

- Sing your material along with the tune until you've found the pocket, or the rhythm that fits the words, more or less, to the music. Sing it several times.

- Now, practice your composition regularly until you've got it memorized.

- Prepare to remember this strange marriage of music and words until your dying day—whether you want to or not.

Kids: Developmental Listening

The first ten years of children's relationship with music can be broken down into developmental stages:

- **Birth to one year:** Newborns like soothing music and the sound of the human voice—preferably Mom's. Sing lullabies to soothe your baby, upbeat songs to stimulate her. Rattles, blocks, music boxes, and musical mobiles can all spur your baby's curiosity and inspire him to explore the world of sound.

- **1-2:** Now the body enters the picture, and one-year-olds can experiment with clapping and moving body parts to music. This is a kinesthetic tune-up that could enhance coordination over the long term, so spend some regular time listening and moving to music.

- **2-3:** At two, kids can move their entire bodies to music, walking, running, bouncing, swaying, nodding their heads, and tapping their feet. It's also time to start singing—imperfect, partial phrases of favorite songs.

- **3-4:** Start piano lessons—as well as singing along to favorite recordings. Children this age are forging neural networks to encode melodies, so encourage them to sing their favorite songs from memory. Don't worry if they're out of tune—they probably will be. The point is to help mold the young, plastic cortex for better lifetime cognition. Music is also a social undertaking for three-year-olds, so encourage group listening and singing, as well as playing games and acting out to music.

- **4-5:** This is the silly stage, so stock up on funny songs to listen to and encourage your four-year-old to make up his own wacky tunes. These kids are also starting to get rhythm. Drums, clappers, sticks, and shakers are good play-along instruments to have on hand. Five-year-olds start to prefer harmonic consonance and regular rhythms over dissonance and nonmetric music. The age for this development has lowered over the century, from nine in 1910 to five in 1985. Researchers attribute the change to the influence of simple, predictable music in mass media; it certainly suggests the profound and early influence of cultural conditioning on musical tastes.

- **6-9:** This age marks the ability to distinguish between different sounds. Try pointing out the drum, voice, and other sounds in the music you listen to, and encourage your child to identify them herself. Age seven appears to be when full-blown music perception really begins, and the development of rhythmic and tonal skills now may determine musical aptitude—and other cognitive operations—for life. Surround your seven- to nine-year-old with a richness of music in a variety of styles, and encourage her to sing and play along both with the music and by herself.

- **10:** It's all over now. Your child will be quite sure that she knows what she likes and nothing you say can make any difference. So be sure to foresee age ten; introduce your child to the joys and cognitive benefits of quality music during the formative years that precede it.[40]

For recommended kids' listening by age group, see Jill Jarnow's *All Ears: How to Choose and Use Recorded Music for Children* (Viking Penguin).

Kids: Play It Again, Sam

Children often like to listen to their favorite tunes over and over again, sometimes driving their parents over the brink in the process. But what sounds like endless repetition to you is *learning*—the creation and reinforcement of neural codes—to your child. Repeated listening allows children to master the language, melody, rhythm, and imagery of songs, which is good for both their cognitive and psychological development.

Buy yourself some patience with a portable tape player your child can listen to on his own. You might want to consider a Walkman-style player with headphones—maybe even one for each child before your next car trip. Teach your children to keep the volume low enough that they can hear you talking through their headphones.[41]

Kids: Quality

You want the best for your children, and evidence suggests that the best music for their cognitive development is classical or other complex music, and folk-type songs with a variety of interesting instruments and meaningful lyrical content. So how to steer them in this direction if they're stuck on Barney or Ice Cube? Develop a strategic listening policy:

- Start off with a favorite song to put your young listener in a receptive mood. Match the music's energy level to your child's.

- Follow with the music you want to introduce. Forget Chopin if he's running and jumping—try a Sousa march instead.

- Share the listening experience with your child. Smile, dance, sing, and provide all the positive reinforcement in your parental power.

- Settle for less. If your child resists, play just one track and promise to go back to the favorite. Don't push or insist, but do persist. Preferences are temporary, but lifelong tastes sneak up on kids when they're not looking.[42]

A Houseful of Music

Remember: Your music tunes your child's brain just as it does yours. So if you're cranking up Bruce Springsteen while your husband is trying to put the kids to bed, don't be surprised when your evening is interrupted by energetic, restless children.

Brainwork

In the Salt Mines of the Mind

So music is great for the cognitive development of kids, but what if you're a grown-up beyond hope of cortical reorganization, just hoping to keep your mind on your work? And what if your workday lasts longer than the fifteen minutes of a Mozart dose?

There is musical hope for the daily brainwork of adults. First, the latest-breaking news from the Salk Institute for Biological Studies: Experiments with mice indicate that even adults can add brain cells and system capacity to key areas of the brain *if they receive enough neurological stimulus*—and music should certainly fill that bill.[43] This 1997 study was the first to contradict the belief that all neurological enhancement ceases after early childhood, and it supports the case for applying the braintuning techniques in this chapter throughout your life.

Beyond its neural priming and memory-pumping power, music can also, without adding a single brain cell, help keep you on task as you try to accomplish your daily job.

Cathy is a librarian. Unlike most guardians of those hushed, tomblike rooms, she plays classical music all day long, and gets frequent comments from her customers about how much they like the music and the atmosphere it creates. Meanwhile, the musical stimulation helps to keep Cathy's reference and research skills sharp during long, high-pressure days.

"I put it on for myself at first," Cathy says. "I don't care if libraries are traditionally silent—there's just no way I can work all day without music. But when the positive comments started to roll in, I realized I'd enhanced the working environment for my customers."

This library's users, it turns out, are the high-powered financiers of one of the nation's major international banks. Cathy's defiance of library protocol has made her DJ to some of the biggest-money decisions in the world.

Listening to Focusing music while you work has been shown to induce a more dedicated and concentrated mood.[44] It can regulate your brain waves to produce the alpha frequencies you need for concentration or the beta waves that encourage active mental attention.[45] Music can add energy to your efforts by increasing your physiological arousal, or it can improve your performance by alleviating task anxiety.[46] It can also increase your attention span and speed your pace to help you work faster and longer.[47] And music's elegant structure, mathematical basis, and orderly progress through time can organize and drive your thoughts through a long workday.

Working Under Pressure

David, a freshly minted lawyer, was working on a case that a senior associate had hinted would determine whether he'd be asked to stay on at the firm. David was swimming in a sea of depositions, research, and briefs—and every time he sat down to piece them together, his mind froze, paralyzed with fear. What if he misinterpreted a ruling? Missed a piece of evidence or a precedent? Misused legal language? David passed his days picking up and putting down pieces of paper. His brief remained unwritten.

One day in the firm's library, David spotted a fellow second-year—a fast-tracker who everyone agreed was partnership material. She was wearing a Walkman and eating Maalox while she worked.

David took his cue and dashed out at lunch to buy a Walkman and a collection of Pat Metheny tapes. He came back, sat down, and strapped on his headphones. After a minute or two of musical decompression, David wrote his first words.

Working can be stressful. Whether you hate your job, fear failure, or just freeze up at your desk, work-related stress can hamper your performance.

One of the ways music has been shown to improve task concentration is by alleviating anxiety, freeing you to focus on the job.[48] An experiment involving surgeons found that they performed with greatest speed and accuracy when listening to music of their choice, which was classical for forty-six out of fifty, and which destressed the doctors by lowering their pulse and blood pressure.[49] Focusing or Relaxing music can also quiet your mind when it gets too busy by producing alpha brain waves—best for quiet, focused thinking.[50] Whether you're a surgeon working under operating-room stress, a student taking a test that could make or break your GPA, or a harried professional with an overflowing in-box, music can chill you out for better performance.

Wide-Awake Work

Work-related stress can put you on edge, but then there are also times when, despite your impending deadline, all you want to do is sleep. When you're feeling fatigued, Focusing or Energizing music can help job performance by increasing your physiological arousal level, increasing system capacity and facilitating performance.[51] It also works on your mind, generating the beta waves required for attentive mental activity.[52]

Tina had just graduated from college, gotten her first career-track job, and discovered New York's nightlife. The late-night club scene was an exciting world that introduced her to many contacts in the fashion industry, but mornings on the job were tough as she tried to get up to speed on the complex and detail-oriented work of tracking inventory and orders for a clothing design firm. During the workday, Tina felt like she carried the entire force of gravity on the top of her skull.

Then she took a tip from her high-energy nightlife, where music kept the party going for hours. A boombox on her desk and a mix of reggae and jazz helped keep Tina alert through her double life, and her nighttime networking and daytime diligence paid off with a promotion. She celebrated by taking the night off to catch up on her sleep.

Music can be a substitute for or adjunct to your coffee mug, and is less likely to give you the jitters or develop a case of terminal mold.

Concentration

You're at the computer adding the crucial lines of code to a routine you've been debugging for hours. You've almost finished the string of commands when suddenly you're interrupted by the sound of a loud snore from the cubicle next door. The syntax escapes from your brain into the atmosphere, you've lost your place, and the entire office explodes into a chorus of coughing and sniffling.

Distractions are built into most work environments. Add our natural tendency to let our minds wander toward topics like lunch, bills, boyfriends, and girlfriends, and it's a miracle we get anything done at all. In such a situation, Focusing music can screen out noise to save the day.

Speed and Efficiency

With some tasks, your goal is simply to dispatch them as quickly and efficiently as possible. Music with a brisk tempo has been shown to make people read faster[53]—and it might push your pace in other tasks, too. Focusing music can help you go longer,[54] extending your attention span until the job is done.

Braintuning Basics: Brain Work

The Concentration Game

When you need to concentrate, the most effective music is the kind you don't really listen to that works subtly in the background so you can focus on your primary task. The most important criterion is steady volume. Next, keep the tempo even. And finally, instrumentation should be as constant as possible, so solo instruments work well. Listen for something as clear and uncluttered as you'd like your mind to be.[56]

Music, Work and Muzak

Many studies have shown that music in the workplace increases productivity, reduces errors, and contributes to employee happiness. Across cultures and throughout time, people have used work songs for everything from driving mules and grinding corn to making automobiles. In fact, it was the industrial workplace that spawned Muzak, which provided relief from the deadening repetition of assembly-line work.[55]

But with no solos, minor keys, pieces longer than three minutes, or dynamic ranges greater than twenty-five decibels (versus fifty on an average recording), Muzak has become an unwelcome cliché in many contemporary workplaces, and it might actually cause fatigue. "I've worked at a lot of places that played elevator music over the PA," said a survey respondent. "And that often made me tired and made work more difficult."

Is there a postindustrial Muzak? What does work music sound like in the age of the Internet? Muzak was designed as a kind of Prozac for the ears, but do you really want to be serene and dumbly mellow while you work?

Music might literally tune your brain for workplace performance. Explore the possibilities in this chapter—and stay tuned for further developments in this exciting field.

Boot Up Your Brain

What's the first thing most desk workers do to kick off the working day? Boot up their computers. This moment initiates all the production that follows until you power down at night, so you want the mood to be right.

If your computer has a sound card, set the tone for your day by programming some braintuning music into your boot routine. Pick a brief energizing motif that makes you feel motivated and bright. Carmen, a media buyer, prefers the theme from *Rocky*. Change the music for new phases—when you take on a new account, get a promotion, switch bosses, or after any unpleasant developments on the job that give the excerpt negative associations.

Instant Tune-Ups

Feeling a little rusty in the middle of a good work streak? Stop for a moment and follow the Focusing music you have playing. Pick out the individual parts, then pay attention to how they interrelate. Listen to how each phrase develops, resolves, and then begins again. Then turn back to your work and emulate the brilliant structure and form that is music.

Calm and Clear

When stress steals your concentration, calm down by taking a moment to listen to Focusing or Relaxing music. Keep the music on in the background when you return to work.

Look Lively

Music can also recharge you on the job when your batteries run low:

- If you've got a serious case of drowsies, begin with a musical alertness break (see chapter 1, Energize), then continue with background music that perks along at a steady pace. Think of the music as a pacesetter for your work.

- Though Energizing music makes a good break, it's bad background for mental work.[1] Getting too aroused tends to distract you, triggers stress, and makes you want to move your body more than your mind. If you find yourself fidgeting or impatient, change your music to something slower and more relaxed.

Ear Blinders

Headphones rule among tools for focusing your mind. They've even been found to help people with attention deficit disorder concentrate on their work. In addition to blocking out distracting sounds, headphones provide a direct energy feed to your brain. They also prevent the braintuning upper frequencies from getting sucked up by the carpet and curtains. Use headphones and Focusing music to:

- Screen out noise from your surroundings.

- Discourage chatty coworkers who like to gossip just when you kick into high gear.

- Inject music right into your mind, like a stereophonic thinking cap. But beware—distracting music will be even more detrimental to your concentration at such close range. Choose carefully.

Speed Racer

When you're cataloguing, coding, running programs, skimming text for keywords, formatting documents, filing, or anything else you'd like to dispatch quickly:

- Choose fast but nondistracting music to energize your efforts.

- You should feel pushed but not stressed. If the music is much faster than your work pace, you won't feel efficient—just out of synch.

Ramp: Real-Music Muzak

One of the tricks to Muzak programming is its fifteen-minute build cycle.[58] To keep your attention, each selection is slightly faster and louder, denser, or busier than the one before (remember the iso principle from previous chapters?). Because you can only build for so long before you're blasting speed metal through the office and people are banging their heads on their desks, you drop the intensity back to base level every fifteen minutes and begin again.

The so-called *ramp archetype* of a slow incremental buildup of stimulus followed by a sudden drop and repetition of the process has proven effective for prolonging attention in a variety of settings.[59] Take advantage of Muzak's extensive productivity research without embracing the company's aesthetic limitations by making your own ramp tape:

- Choose a fifteen-minute sequence of selections that gradually increase in volume, tempo, and ensemble size or intensity.

- Prevent monotony by using a staggered tempo build. For instance, begin with sixty beats per minute, drop to fifty, jump up to seventy-five, back off to seventy, and so on.

- Vary the rhythm of selections by listening for whether the beats fall into groups of two, three, or four, then alternate pieces of different rhythmic groupings throughout the sequence.

- Remember that this is a gradual, subtle build. If you end up with Slayer at minute ten, you know you've gone too far.

- Tape fifteen minutes of silence after each ramp sequence, or simply turn off the tape for a while. The alternation of music and silence helps keep you stimulated.

- Start and finish each fifteen-minute sequence at a slightly higher intensity level (louder and faster) than the one before, building the block sequence into the productivity troughs of your day. Muzak research pinpoints the low points for office workers at eleven A.M. to noon and three to four P.M.; adjust as necessary to your own schedule and biorhythms. Remember that the increments should be slight, and drop the base level back down after each trough.

The net effect of your ramps should be something like drinking stronger and stronger coffee as the day goes on—but without the shakes or insomnia.

The Single-Disc Method

If making your own ramp tape or programming your CD player is more than you can fathom, try a simpler, more extended version with your CD player or Discman:

- Select two groups of three CDs, one for the morning and one for the afternoon. Each group should build in intensity—for example, a disc of solo piano, then some Bach concertos, and finally some smooth jazz.

- Play each group of discs in order of intensity into your morning and afternoon troughs. Take fifteen minutes of silence between each one to refresh your mind.

Motivation

Music As Pavlovian Cue

I received my undergraduate education to a soundtrack of carillon bells. Hourly chimes woke the student body from the daze of one class and sent us scurrying across the Dartmouth Green to the next. Each bell tower mini-concert was a call to intellectual arms, the piercing vibration of seventeen bells tuning up our brains to the electrical capacity necessary to learning and the pursuit of excellence.

It must have worked. The college maintains the highest academic standards despite its students' reputation for favoring bonhomie over braininess.

The Dartmouth carillon bells were recently reprogrammed to expand the repertoire beyond the "Alma Mater" and "Dartmouth Undying" to include Madonna, the Beatles, and TV themes. The neurological implications of the new repertoire remain untested, but the implication seems clear: a Pavlovian cue is whatever makes you drool.

Music's mood-inducing power can be a great motivator when you sit down to work. In addition to encouraging concentration in general, a certain musical style or recording can become associated with a particular project or type of work in your mind. Hearing it, just like Pavlov and his bells, makes you want to do the job.

It's also been proven that if you learn something while listening to a certain type of music, playing that music can enhance your recall of the material later on.[60] So, when the scope of your project requires that you attack it in several smaller work sessions, music can provide a thread of cognitive continuity that immediately recalls past discoveries as you face the next phase. This can help when you feel like you're backpedaling on a big undertaking—and who at some point hasn't?

Andy wrote his master's thesis by playing the soundtrack from *The Piano* every time he sat down to work. The music always returned him to the mind-set of the project—the longest thing he'd ever written—and reminded him of what he'd been thinking about last time.

Jenna, an academic researcher in education, says that she, too, listens to *The Piano* every time she sits down to code one of her data-gathering interviews—a demanding analytical task that she hates. "I always know when Jenna is coding," says her husband. "I hear *that song*—and I know to steer clear." For Jenna, who would rather think great thoughts than gather the data that supports them, the music is both relief from the repetition and reward for buckling down to this painful but necessary task.

Keith, a screenwriter, says that he finds inspiration in listening to movie soundtracks while he writes. "Picture all these geeky screenwriters typing away to pieces with titles like 'Edward Scissorhands Goes Shopping,' " says Keith.

The sound of your mood music might vary from one project or task to the next, but once you've attached it to your opus magnus, chances are that you can trigger your motivation with the flick of a CD switch.

Reward

Jenna has another trick to conquer her aversion to coding. For each interview she completes, she compensates herself with a song by her favorite group of the moment. "For awhile, I was using cookies as reward," says Jenna. "Ultimately, that wasn't going to work. A song by Smashing Pumpkins is what I work for now."

In addition to triggering the mood to return to an ongoing project, music can serve as a reward for good work. This can help keep you focused in a world in which rewards are rare. If your paycheck is just a tool to keep your landlord off your back or if you're disappointed that they don't give good grades in the real world, you might find yourself wondering, "What am I working for?" Some people turn to food, drugs, or alcohol as payback. Music exacts a lower price.

Musical rewards have been shown to help talkative students quiet down in class. They can make people complain less. Whatever your challenges, *contingent presentation* of music—listening as a reward for productive behavior—can motivate your efforts and improve your results.[61]

Braintuning Basics: Motivation

I'm in the Mood to Work

- Match your music to the nature of the task—maybe electronic music if you're making semiconductors, or Peruvian flutes to write your Spanish paper.

- Play the same music from one work session to the next to enhance your memory of what you did and learned in previous sessions.

Musical Payback

Give yourself a musical treat for a job well done:

- Pick a particular style or artist you love, and reserve those recordings for rewards when you've completed a task. Don't listen without earning the right! Like rich chocolate desserts, it won't be a treat if you indulge all the time.

- Match the music with how you want to feel upon completion. Try something Energizing (chapter 1) if you're fatigued and need to recharge. A Relaxing selection (chapter 2) can soothe you if you're stressed. Uplifting music (chapter 5) has a celebratory sound—or just enjoy your personal favorite.

The Focus Music-Mood Checklist*

❑ Steady, deliberate pulse (sixty beats per minute recommended by some experts)

❑ Simple, predictable rhythms (4/4 time)

*This checklist is for background learning and working music. See the discography that follows for further discussion of the complex music that can prime neural networks.

❑ Symmetrical form and phrasing

❑ Clearly defined phrases of short to moderate length

❑ Familiar sounds that you like

❑ Major key

❑ No lyrics

❑ Integrated ensemble and texture

❑ Transparent texture you can think through

❑ High frequencies (strings)

❑ Dry tones without excessive reverberation

❑ Constant volume

❑ Elegant, virtuosic performance

❑ Instrumental attack

Avoid unfamiliar sounds, distracting lyrics, deep sounds or heavy bass, demanding music that can create a dual task paradigm, or selections that stir up strong emotions.[62]

Test Your Focus Factor

This chapter covers situations requiring some very different cognitive skills, so you shouldn't be surprised if you require different types of music to work at your peak in contrasting settings. In fact, you should fully expect an engaging snippet of Mozart to prime you better for a math problem than for a reading session.

The best strategy is to test your response to Focusing music in the different thought and work challenges you encounter, and compile separate lists of your favorites for each. See page 24 in the introduction for instructions on testing and recording your music-mood response. A Focus discography follows the quiz. Start by testing your favorite styles from the list and recording your results in the journal that follows.

The Focus Music-Mood Test

	Before Listening	After Listening	Change, Before to After
I Feel	(1–5)	(1–5)	(+ or –, 0–4)
Sharp	_____	_____	_____
Capable	_____	_____	_____
Interested	_____	_____	_____
Clear	_____	_____	_____
Focused	_____	_____	_____
Analytical	_____	_____	_____
Motivated	_____	_____	_____
Logical	_____	_____	_____
Quick	_____	_____	_____
Present	_____	_____	_____
Total Change: Your Focus Factor (0–40)			_____

The Focus Music-Mood Journal

Date	Situation	Selection	Score
_____	_____	_____	_____
_____	_____	_____	_____
_____	_____	_____	_____
_____	_____	_____	_____
_____	_____	_____	_____
_____	_____	_____	_____
_____	_____	_____	_____
_____	_____	_____	_____
_____	_____	_____	_____
_____	_____	_____	_____
_____	_____	_____	_____
_____	_____	_____	_____
_____	_____	_____	_____
_____	_____	_____	_____
_____	_____	_____	_____
_____	_____	_____	_____
_____	_____	_____	_____
_____	_____	_____	_____

Braintuning Music: Focus

Even among people of many different tastes, classical seems to be the Focusing music of choice—perhaps because we associate this type of music with a cultivated mind. The Focus discography reflects this preference, but also broadens the possibilities into the great musical world beyond. New sounds could expand your mind.

Western Classical

Complex music is the proven prescription for neural priming, so if abstract reasoning is what you're after, cue up some **Western orchestral music of the classical era**. Mozart's music has passed the clinical test, but his contemporaries share many of his musical attributes—so why not also try Haydn, C.P.E. Bach, or early Beethoven when you're looking for a right-brain boost?

But if you'd rather aim music's firepower at neurons on the left side of the brain, **19th and 20th-century composers who use complicated rhythms** could light up that part of your mind for language and logical tasks. Ravel, Stravinsky, and Ives all had surprising ways of working with time.

It's striking how many people instinctually choose Baroque music for their brain work even without knowing any of the theories of how it might help them think or remember. The accelerated learning school advocates Baroque compositions emphasizing **stringed instruments** like violin, guitar, mandolin, and harpsichord (as most music of the era does), asserting that the harmonics of high strings help trigger your learning and memory response.

The harpsichord is a true power tool for the mind. A predecessor to the piano whose hammers actually pluck a string each time you press a key, this stately instrument strums away at your brain, insistent and inspiring.

When it comes to the Baroque, **Bach** is king—and was himself given to showing off his intellect. He wrote "The Well-Tempered Clavier" to prove his ability to work in all twenty-four keys, an unprecedented compositional feat. "The Art of the Fugue" covered every fugal form known to mankind. One of Bach's final works, "A Musical Offering," takes a single, simple theme and develops it with various types of counterpoint into thirteen different pieces. It makes that little marketing problem you're grappling with sound easy.

Many other Baroque composers can add a sense of symmetry and structure to your work. Albinoni, Corelli, Couperin, Rameau, Scarlatti, Telemann, and Vivaldi all deserve a place in your desktop collection.

World Classical

Or you can light up your cortex with other world classical traditions—**Indian ragas, Balinese gamelan, Cambodian court music**, or **Middle Eastern orchestras**.

The **Karnatic music of South India** combines composition with improvisation in the complex *ragas* (melodic structures) and *talas* (rhythmic cycles) of Indian art music. Unlike the sometimes-meditative music of the North, Karnatic compositions tend to move at a lively clip, which might be better for neural priming. Players trade phrases and develop ideas in a way that relates to Western art music—but with the added challenge of improvisation.

On the Indonesian island of Bali, the modern *"kebyar"* style of *gamelan* (an orchestra of gongs, xylophones, flutes, and drums) grew out of an ancient tradition in the 1920s and originally, like most classical music styles of the world, was performed to entertain the members of the court. Played with unpadded mallets, *kebyar* means "to burst into flame," describing its virtuosic nature and what will happen to your neurons when you listen. The cyclical build-ups also provide a "ramp" effect. It was hearing a gamelan performance at the 1889 Exposition Universelle in Paris that convinced composer Claude Debussy that the human brain could comprehend harmonies outside of the usual Western scheme and led to his subsequent harmonic experimentation; the strange tunings of the Indonesian scale will certainly activate brain cells as your cortex tries to categorize new pitch relations.

The royal palace tradition of **Cambodia** includes dance and music performed by a ***pinn peat*** ensemble of xylophones, gongs, *sralai thomm* (a bass oboe), drums, and cymbals. The sound is similar to the Balinese *gamelan* but more delicate—and very rare, since the 1970 overthrow of the monarchy threw the tradition into crisis, and few recordings have been made.

Other Instrumental Traditions

Many other instrumental styles can add regular rhythm and sonic pleasure to your work day.

Solo piano often features a steady, understated pulse and a tight dynamic range to keep your mind moving.

The **Japanese *koto*** is a plucked string instrument, something like an

Eastern echo of the harpsichord. Its repertoire, both solo and ensemble, is structured and elegant.

The musical style favored by the "Wave"-type radio stations that are popular in many workplace settings is jazz of a certain pace, tonality, and texture. Whatever your feeling about the Wave format, stations featuring **smooth jazz** are topping Arbitron ratings across the nation. The style seems to make people feel good at work, simultaneously taking the edge off stress and providing enough of a beat to keep listeners feeling lively. By programming your own you can stick to instrumentals and avoid distracting lyrics.

Mood Music

And then there's any kind of music that puts you in the right mood for the job. This is a subjective and personal choice. Just be careful not to diminish your performance by secretly using music as a distraction from work you don't want to do! (See also chapter 7, Create, for a variety of musical styles that might trigger the mood of your project.)

The Braintuning Discography: Focus

STYLE	TITLE
	MELODICALLY & HARMONICALLY COMPLEX MUSIC FOR RIGHT-BRAIN NEURAL PRIMING

Classical Orchestra

- C.P.E. Bach:
- *Concerto for Two Harpsichords Wq. 46.* Gustav Leonhardt and the Collegium Aureum, Deutsche Harmonia Mundi 77061. The 2-keyboard concerto should simulate the effect of the Mozart test piece—but with the extra high harmonics of the harpsichord.
- *6 Symphonies, Wq. 182.* Christopher Hogwood, Academy of Ancient Music, L'Oiseau-Lyre 417124.
- Ludwig van Beethoven. *Symphonies No. 1 and 2.* Herbert von Karajan & the Berlin Philharmonic, Deutsche Grammophon 439001.
- Franz Joseph Haydn:
- *Symphonies No. 94, 100, and 101.* RCA Victor 62564.
- *Symphonies No. 42, 45 (Farewell) and 46.* Trevor Pinnock & the English Concert, Archiv 447281.
- Wolfgang Amadeus Mozart:
- *Sonata for Two Pianos in D Major (K. 488).* Murray Perahia and Radu Lupu, Sony Classical 39511. The actual recording used in the UC-Irvine experiment.
- *Clarinet Concerto in A Major, K. 622.* David Shifrin and the

Mostly Mozart Orchestra, Delos 3020. Performed on a special extended-range clarinet for which the work was originally written, this concerto could expand the range of your mind.

• *Symphonies Nos. 35-41.* Carl Böhm & the Berlin Philharmonic, Deutsche Grammophon 447416. Take your pick from six symphonies.

Middle Eastern Orchestra	• Hassan Erraji. "Hammouda" on *Trance Planet.* Triloka 7206. The sparkling conversation between the *'ud* (lute), *qanun* (hammered zither), and drums is sure to light a fire in your mind.
Balinese Kebyar Gamelan	• Gamelan Semar Pegulingan. *Music of Bali.* Lyrichord 7408. The instruments and temple in which they're played are more than 400 years old..
Cambodian Court Music	• Sam-Ang Sam Ensemble. *Echoes from the Palace: Court Music of Cambodia.* Music of the World 140. High-frequency bell tones and precise melodies and rhythms make a potent and precious elixir for the mind.
South Indian Karnatic Music	• *Vadya Lahari* featuring A. Kanyakumari. Music of the World 125. The viloin in the leading role might remind you of Mozart—but its unusual pairing with the *nadaswaram,* a huge, ear-opening, Indian oboe, definitely won't. The rhythmic complexity of these pieces might also help their neural priming effect cross over into your left brain.

RHYTHMICALLY COMPLEX MUSIC FOR LEFT-BRAIN NEURAL PRIMING

• Mustapha Tettey Addy. *Master Drummer from Ghana.* Lyrichord 7250. Talking drum in the polyrhythmic tradition of West Africa.

• Charles Ives. *Symphony No. 2, Symphony No. 3, Central Park in the Dark.* Leonard Bernstein & the New York Philharmonic Orchestra, Sony Classical 47568.

• Ivo Papasov. *Balkanology.* Hannibal 1363. Bulgarian wedding music gone mad.

• Maurice Ravel. *Daphne et Chloe Suite No. 2.* Paul Paray & the Detroit Symphony Orchestra, Mercury Living Presence 34306. This ballet's unexpected rhythms make it notoriously hard to dance to; sounds like good exercise for your mind.

• Trichy Sankaran. *Laya Vinyas.* Music of the World 120. In India, listeners demonstrate that they can follow the complex *talas,* or rhythmic cycles, with a set of standard hand gestures. Test your own rhythmic IQ with the *mrdangam,* or South Indian drum.

• Igor Stravinsky. *Symphony in 3 Movements.* Columbia Symphony Orchestra, Columbia 42434.

WORK & LEARNING MUSIC

Baroque Strings & Keyboard

• Tomaso Albinoni. *Adagio in G Minor*. Herbert von Karajan & the Berlin Philharmonic, Deutsche Grammophon 413309. Try this for accelerated learning; pieces by Bach, Pachelbel, and Vivaldi on this disc will also do the job.

• Johann Sebastian Bach:

The Art of the Fugue. Harmonia Mundi 901169.

6 Brandenburg Concertos BWV 1046-1051. Trevor Pinnock, The English Concert, Archiv 423492.

6 Cello Suites. Mischa Maisky, Deutsche Grammophon 445373. Try the deep resonance of solo cello when your eardrums are singed by too many high harmonics. Exuberant and driving.

A Musical Offering BWV 1079. Davitt Moroney, Harmonia Mundi 901260. Building on a theme by his patron, the Prussian King Frederick, Bach improvised this piece on the spot, then went home to write it down.

Orchestral Suites 1&2; Concerto for Two Harpsichords BWV 1060 and *Orchestral Suites 3&4; Concerto for Two Harpsichords BWV 1062*. Christopher Hogwood, the Academy of Ancient Music, L'Oiseau Lyre 443181 and 443182. Maybe Bach's Concertos for Two Harpsichords are to your work day what Mozart's Sonata for Two Pianos is to your IQ.

The Well-Tempered Clavier. Davitt Moroney, harpsichord, Harmonia Mundi 1901285. Containing a piece for every existing key, both major and minor, this mental masterpiece proved that the "tempered" scale could work and made possible harmony as we know it now.

• Arcangelo Corelli. *6 Concerti Grossi Op. 6 #7–12*. Nicholas McGegan, Philharmonia Baroque Orchestra, Harmonia Mundi 907015.

• George Frideric Handel:

Concerti Grossi. Orpheus Chamber Orchestra, Deutsche Grammophon 447733. Orchestral dialogues by a Baroque master.

3 Suites ("Water Music"), HWV 348-350, Archiv 410525.

Fitzwilliam Virginal Book Excerpts. Ton Koopman, Capriccio 10211.

Harpsichord music from the famed 17th-century British collection.

The Harmonious Blacksmith. Trevor Pinnock, Deutsche Grammophon 413591. With a title that suggests achieving near-impossible feats on the job, this recording includes harpsichord works by Couperin, Rameau, Bach, and Handel.

• Jean-Philippe Rameau. *Pieces de Clavecin 1724. Nouvelles*

Suites 1728. Harmonia Mundi 1901120 and 1901121. The composer was also an accomplished music theorist and living proof of music's potential benefit to your brain cells.

• Domenico Scarlatti. *19 Sonatas for Harpsichord*. Colin Tilney, Dorian 90103.

• Georg Phillip Telemann. *Vol. 1: La Changeante*. Simon Standage & Collegium Musicum 90, Chandos 0519. Five concertos and an orchestral suite feature the braintuning high harmonics of the violin.

• Antonio Vivaldi:

The Four Seasons (4 Concertos Op. 8 #1–4). Gil Shaham & the Orpheus Chamber Orchestra, Deutsche Grammophon 439933.

Vivaldi Guitar Concertos. Deutsche Grammophon 429528.

Other Solo Keyboard	• Michael Nyman. *The Piano*. Virgin 88274. Not strictly solo, but with nice minimalist drive. • *Piano Solos* and *First Light: Piano Solos*. Narada 61031 and 61059. Good for stressful work—solo piano pieces in a New Age vein keep you calm but also keep you going with steady rhythm and attack. • George Winston. *Summer*. Windham Hill 11107. By an artist who has helped define contemporary solo piano performance.
Japanese Koto	• *Japanese Koto Consort*. Lyrichord 7205. The plucked Japanese lute is delicate and precise.
Smooth Jazz	• Michael Brecker. *Tales from the Hudson*. GRP 191. With Pat Metheny, McCoy Tyner, and Jack DeJohnette. • The Modern Jazz Quartet. *Blues on Bach*. Atlantic 1652. Jazz goes Baroque; the vibraphone is a mini mind massage. • Herbie Hancock. *Maiden Voyage*. Capitol 46339. Instrumental jazz circa 1965. • Pat Metheny. *Question and Answer*. Geffen 24293. • David Sanborn. *A Change of Heart*. Warner Brothers 25479. Breezy alto sax and slick production. • Spyro Gyra. *Heart of the Night*. GRP 9842. Jazz with a light pop flavor.
Instructional Songs	• They Might Be Giants. "James K. Polk" on *Factory Showroom*. Elektra 61862. Quirky rockers tell all about the 11th U.S. president. • *Schoolhouse Rock*. Kid Rhino 72455. An anthology of the original '70s songs. • *Schoolhouse Rock Rocks*. Lava/Atlantic 92681. A Gen-X take on the theme featuring the Lemonheads, Blind Melon, and more.
Singalong Tunes	• Georges Bizet. *Carmen*. Sir Georg Solti, London Philharmonic, London 414489.

• George Frideric Handel. The "Hallelujah Chorus" on *Messiah: Favorite Choruses and Arias*. Robert Shaw & the Atlanta Symphony Orchestra, Telarc 80103.

• Peter Ilyich Tchaikovsky. *Nutcracker Suite*. London 417300.

• John Philip Sousa. *Original All-American Sousa*. Delos 3102.

• "Tequila," "The Twelve Days of Christmas," "Yankee Doodle," or your own favorite tune.

Mood Music	• Ludwig van Beethoven. Second movement of *Symphony No. 7*. Carlos Klieber & the Vienna Philharmonic, Deutsche Grammophon 447400. An insistent pulsing question, a slow build in intensity, and a few moments of majesty to awaken and inspire you. • Wolfgang Amadeus Mozart. Second movement of *Symphony No. 38* on *Symphonies 35–41*. Carl Böhm and the Berlin Philharmonic, Deutsche Grammophon 447416. Steady and stately, this should trigger an organized state of mind. • Pink Floyd. *The Wall*. Columbia 36183. Its familiarity improved recall and attention among teenage boys.
Alpha Brain-waves Sound	• Dr. Jeffrey Thompson. *Brainwave Suite: Alpha*. Relaxation Company 3051. Sound pulses said to create alpha waves, associated with concentration and meditative states. Accompanied by guitar, shakuhachi flute, and nature sounds.

See page 255 for Sources.

Focus: The Braintuning 5

A diverse sampling from the discography to get you started:

• Wolfgang Amadeus Mozart. *Sonata for Two Pianos in D Major (K. 488)*. Murray Perahia and Radu Lupu, Sony Classical 39511.

• *Vadya Lahari* featuring A. Kanyakumari. Music of the World 125.

• Johann Sebastian Bach. *The Well-Tempered Clavier*. Davitt Moroney, harpsichord, Harmonia Mundi 90185.

• Antonio Vivaldi. *The Four Seasons (4 Concertos Op. 8 #1–4)*. Gil Shaham & the Orpheus Chamber Orchestra, Deutsche Grammophon 439933.

• *Japanese Koto Consort*. Lyrichord 7205.

Music Makes Me Compos Mentis

Beware of the wrong working music! When you hear a husky-voiced singer crooning a sensuous melody in Portuguese, you will want a warm beach and a cool piña colada—not a computer and an in-box.

Instead, follow the suggestions in this chapter for music that stimulates your mind. Feel your neurons fire up as the first sweet strains of electrical energy flow through your cortex.

Remember also to save your Focusing repertoire for mental efforts. Mixing it up with memories of celebrations or erotic ecstasy could wreak havoc on your work day. Associate these sounds with your mind's finest moments, and all the natural neurological benefits of music will be yours.

Four

Heal

Proto-doctor Hippocrates knew all about the healing power of music, but the history of music as medicine goes back much farther, all the way to the Kahum papyrus, the oldest known written account of medical practices. Today, as the national health care crisis begs for alternative solutions, doctors and nurses are using music in clinics, hospitals, and hospices to facilitate treatment, control pain, and heal. Take a tip from the length of medical history and let music help keep you well and weather the traumas of being sick.

Heal Overview

Healing Music Can Help You With:	Use These Techniques if You Are:	How Music Helps:
Immunity	Thinking preventively—stop germs in their tracks; facing flu season or a local epidemic; committed to long-term wellness.	Activates a neuroendocrine mechanism in the limbic system to boost beneficial hormones and blood cells and suppress harmful ones.

Illness & Injury	Sick or hurt, from a tension headache to a heart attack.	Lowers blood pressure and heart and respiratory rates as it boosts mood—both important to recovery, even survival.
Pain	Submitting to the speculum, needle, tube, bronchoscope, dentist's drill, or other invader; suffering pain from an illness or injury.	Acts as an "audioanalgesic" to raise your pain threshold, lessen pain's sensation, and reduce stress symptoms.
Surgery	Going under the knife or in recovery.	Reduces preoperative anxiety and eases postoperative pain; prevents posttraumatic stress disorder by blocking surgical sounds and reducing stress signals; stimulates muscles for recuperative therapy.
Maternity	Pregnant or in labor.	Provides rhythm and mood-altering effect to help reduce anxiety, pace breathing, relax muscles, reduce perceived pain, and personalize the experience.
Sick Children	Dealing with the double blow of relinquishing a child in pain to the hospital.	Works on a nonverbal level to reduce a child's fear and distress, increase expression and cooperation, and ease pain with lower doses of drugs.
Aging; Death and Dying	Coping with depression, Alzheimer's, or other age-related illness; dealing with the grieving and physical pain of terminal illness.	Helps the patient communicate; reduces disruptive or isolating behaviors; increases interest in external events; enhances quality of life.

In the current climate of therapeutic consumerism, it's hard to decide where to put your precious health care time and money. Laser surgery or contact lenses? Antibiotics or homeopathy? A health club membership or home blood pressure kit? It's exciting to have so many options, but it's also confusing, expensive, and sometimes risky. In your wellness toolbox, music can be an easy and low-cost contributor. It's proven effective, both by centuries of use and contemporary clinical studies. It's almost free and has no side effects. And you probably like it a lot better than the average medicine. Hearing is the first sense fully attained by humans (within 135 days after conception) and the last one typically lost,[1]—so from the womb to the last breaths of life, you can use sound to enhance your health.

At Kaiser Permanente in California, music is used to prep patients for surgery and chemotherapy and to help treat back pain, spinal injuries, high blood pressure, migraines, and ulcers. Other medical facilities from Beth Israel Hospital in Boston to Mount Zion in San Francisco have added music to their roster of treatments.

There's good reason for this recent wave of interest in music's medical applications. An assessment of medical music research studies conducted in the 1980s showed that music had a significant impact on (in order of effectiveness):[2]

- Pulse rate (undue elevation of which can cause medical distress)
- Amount of pain medication required
- Perceived or observed pain
- Muscle relaxation
- Perceived or observed anxiety
- Stress hormone levels
- Blood pressure
- Mood and attitude
- Motor ability
- Length of labor in childbirth

These studies also found that music improved walking speed, exhalation strength, physical comfort, length of hospitalization, and satisfaction and contentment among patients undergoing medical treatment, as well as increasing movement and weight gain for newborn babies.

In a recent survey of German medical students, music ranked high as a treatment adjunct, reflecting what the researcher calls a shift toward "biopsychosocial" thinking among medical practitioners.[3] This is borne out by a four-year study at a German hospital, which found that both listening to and participating in music was a useful adjunct to internal medicine for a wide variety of illnesses.[4]

As cost pressures and changing attitudes shift more direct-care responsibilities from doctors to nurses, both parties acknowledge the need for interventions that nurses can administer independently.[5] One such treatment is music, and many nurses are embracing it as a tool to manage patients' pain, autonomic indicators, and anxiety. That beats waiting for the doctor to get to you on rounds.

The literature on using music as medicine ranges from early music therapy tracts[6] to ethnographic descriptions[7]; work by contemporary musicians who draw on indigenous and New Age ideas, often to create new compositions for healing[8]; and an extensive body of clinical research published in medical and music therapy journals in recent decades. Most of the research presented in this chapter comes from the field of traditional Western medicine and reflects the scientific method. Because the outcome of such studies is proving music's efficacy to the medical mainstream, increasing numbers of patients are having the opportunity to experience musical treatment, allowing them to draw their own conclusions.

The World of Musical Medicine

You need look no further than Native American culture for a rich tradition of healing with music. The Navajo nation employs music healing ceremonies that can last more than a week. Ojibwa Midewiwin healers have an entire repertoire of songs to treat the sick. If you're a member of the Winnebago nation and lucky enough to own a grizzly bear song, you can allegedly heal wounds by singing it, while the Papago of Arizona cure with songs given to them by the deer, badger, horned toad, rattlesnake, and lizard. The Cherokee people have songs specifically targeted to treat ailments from snakebite to fever.

Other music-healing cultures include the Sufis, who believe that music heals through its effect on the endocrine system—a hypothesis now supported by clinical research. In India, the 10,000-year-old tradition of Ayurvedic healing relies upon Gandharva music, along with therapies that access the other four senses. Chinese healing music is based on theories of balancing *yin* and *yang*, correlating the five tones of the scale with organs in the body.

Music is an integral part of medical practice around the world. As science measures the physiological impact of music on bodily processes affected by illness or injury, it's interesting to see the convergence of Western medicine with non-Western and native practices and gratifying to have rediscovered a time-honored tool for better health care. Whether you're going to the dentist or facing a frightening diagnosis, music can help you heal, manage your pain, and cope with the ramifications of being ill.

Health for the Whole Self

Healing applications of music integrate its physiological and psychological effects to attain desired states in the body (usually alleviating physical stress symptoms) while it provides emotional comfort and distraction for your mind. Whether regulating your hormones, your heartbeat, or your imagery, music can target the places where healing occurs as effectively as some more intrusive therapies.

For that reason, many holistic health care professionals advocate using music as part of an integrated treatment plan. Holistic practitioners treat the entire person—the mind-body system that is tangibly linked by the production of hormones. Patients like the noninvasive, natural form of such treatments, the sense of control they gain over their health, and the individualized nature of care.

In holistic terms, health care practitioners say that music can help sick patients:[9]

- Cope with the severity and acuteness of their illness

- Deal with the effects of illness on the individual, family, job, and financial position

- Fight fear, anxiety, and depression

- Remain socially engaged

Immunity

A Metropolitan Life Insurance survey concluded that orchestra conductors live 38 percent longer than the general population.[10] That might be partly because they get a lot more exercise on the job than most of us. But they might also be staying well with music.

Antibodies, helper T cells, killer T cells, suppresser T cells, natural killer cells, lymphocytes, phagocytes, granulocytes, neutrophils, messenger molecules—these cells and molecules are the foot soldiers of your immune system, equipped to defend you against disease. Their levels are governed in part by the health of your emotional, cognitive, and behavioral life—and usually, the more the merrier.

Your immune system's enemies include antigens and pathogens (germs), carcinogens (cancer-causing agents), and stress hormone secretions like adrenaline, cortisone, thyroxin, and endorphin.

The hypothalamus, which helps regulate the secretion of immunity-eating stress hormones, is part of the limbic system, the emotional center of the brain that is also involved in interpreting musical sound. Research suggests that a neuroendocrine mechanism in the hypothalamus provides a link between the music you listen to and the strength of your immune system.[11]

When healthy adults listened to fifteen minutes of music they liked, their blood tests afterwards revealed higher levels of interleukin-1, a polypeptide hormone necessary to immunological reactions, and lower levels of the stress hormone cortisol, both signs of stronger immunity.[12] In a German experiment, a Strauss waltz and a piece by Ravi Shankar lowered blood levels of immunity-attackers cortisol, t-PA antigen, and noradrenaline.[13]

It is this limbic connection between music and hormones that might underlie the belief systems of various indigenous healing musics. The Temiar people of Malaysia, for example, have an elaborate practice that uses music to combat the toxicity of emotions[14]—in other words, to reduce levels of immune-depleting stress hormones. Shaman healers of the Kodi people use drums and gongs to resolve bad feelings between the patient and his relatives, who are thought to have brought his illness upon him.[15] This ritualized access to the limbic system through music could derive its medical power through the neuroendocrine mechanism.

Music also keeps you well by entraining your circadian rhythms. When your biorhythms, as measured by things like body temperature and biochemistry, get out of synch with your schedule, your performance is impaired and your immunity put at risk. Regular music and relaxation sessions have been shown to match up your body temperature, electrolytes (fluid balancers), corticosteroids (hormones), and neurotransmitters (brain chemicals)—your circadian rhythms—with your daily patterns and activities.[16]

Braintuning Basics: Immunity

Love Thyself and Thy Music

In healing applications, music's effect has been observed to be the strongest when patients listen to music they like. Perhaps more than in any other braintuning activity, choosing music you prefer is of paramount importance to the healing process.[17]

To maximize the neuroendocrine impact of Healing music, choose your own. Use portable tape and CD players, and screen out piped-in music with personal headphones.

Take a Chill Pill

You can feed your immune cells and minimize the hormones that destroy them by listening to Healing or Relaxing music (see the discography in this chapter or in chapter 2, Relax) any time you feel wound up in your mind or body. Keep a Walkman close at hand when you're stressed, traveling, undergoing a change in weather or schedule, or any other time you feel susceptible to getting sick. Put on your headphones just like you would pop a pill—but with no worry about interactions, side effects, expense, or addiction.

Get Your Daily Dose

Immunity is an ongoing process that basically boils down to protecting yourself from physical and emotional stresses on a daily basis. A regular music schedule can help keep your immune system functioning at optimum levels just like steady eating, exercise, and sleep patterns. To use music as a preventive tool, schedule listening sessions into your day:

- Try five minutes of Healing music every hour if you have very stressful days; a half hour every evening if you have quiet time then; fifteen minutes at midday—whatever works. The important thing is to establish a pattern and stick with it, just like with your meals and your workouts.

- Expect and look forward to your music break as you would, say, lunch. Think of it as a reward and a self-nurturing time. Also consider it necessary; your circadian rhythms are relying on your musical cue to gear you up or down for what comes next. Your T cells are praying for relief from the cortisol nibbling at their walls. Your adrenal glands are coiling up with each passing nerve impulse, and unless they are soothed with sound, they may strike.

• Take time for some Healing music whenever you feel stressed. What seems like mere anxiety can translate to a literal attack on your physical defenses.

Illness and Injury

When you do get sick or hurt, supporting your immune system with music can help you heal faster. Illness and injury are physically stressful, and the side effects of stress can contribute to a downward spiral in which your already-vulnerable body gets weaker and less able to fight off invaders or heal tissues. By relaxing your body and easing the burden on your heart, arteries, and nerves, music can intercede in this cycle and give your body room to recover.

You can also use Healing music as an easy-access treatment for minor or routine symptoms or procedures. Got a tension headache? When researchers played headache victims their favorite music as a reward for decreased forehead tension (measured by an electromyogram), the subjects willed their heads to relax and decreased their headache activity.[18]

Musical relaxation has been shown to decrease the symptoms of asthma.[19] Listening to music can also reduce anxiety and distract patients during kidney dialysis, making the procedure less uncomfortable.[20]

Or maybe you're sick and tired of being laid up in bed. A Japanese study of patients confined to their beds found that classical music significantly decreased the frequency and intensity of their complaints.[21]

Music is even more useful as your condition gets more serious. A bad illness or wound means higher bodily stress levels—just as you have to submit to the sonic chaos of the hospital.

Many people know firsthand that one of the primary risks of checking into the hospital is getting sicker, and an improperly managed sound environment can contribute to this danger. Florence Nightingale herself noted that sudden, sharp, or unnecessary noise was harmful to patients, but that music, particularly the human voice and soft strings, was a beneficial treatment.[22] Now doctors, nurses, and medical researchers are recognizing sound as an important variable in patient healing that must be as carefully controlled as sterility procedures and treatment protocols.[23]

The EPA recommends that the noise levels in hospitals should be limited to 40 to 45 decibels during the day and 35 decibels at night, but average hospital noise ranges from 57.2 decibels in the postanesthesia recovery unit to 58 to 72 decibels in intensive care.[24] Noise can increase blood levels of the stress hormones adrenaline, cortisol, and ACTH; decrease growth hormone; suppress lymphocyte function (an immune reaction); and worsen inflammations. All these processes impede healing and immunity.

Noise can also increase the need for pain medication. One study showed that the amount of pain medicine dispensed rose when noise levels exceeded fifty decibels—less than in the average hospital.[25]

ER!

In an emergency situation, stabilizing your vital signs can be critical to your survival. Emergency rooms and intensive care units have added music to their array of high-tech equipment because of its power to do just that:

- In one study, patients with acute myocardial infarction (heart attack) decreased their heart rate, respiration rate, and anxiety levels by listening to music with a tempo of sixty beats per minute.[26] In general, music has been shown to have both physiological and psychological benefits for cardiac patients in intensive care.[27]

- Intensive care patients listening to music showed a significant decrease in blood pressure and were found to be more positive on emotional status assessments than fellow patients without music.[28]

- Music can ease the trauma of intubation, the painful first step in mechanical ventilation.[29] It also reduces the ongoing distress of ventilation, as shown by an experiment in which those who listened to music had significantly lower heart and respiratory rates and answered more positively on a mood state assessment than the control group.[30]

- When St. Joseph's Hospital of New York installed Muzak in the intensive care unit, heart attacks dropped and the unit's mortality rate clocked in at 8 to 12 percent below the national average.[31] The effect might have been even greater with music preferred by the patients.

- The machine-based environment of intensive care units often subjects patients to the additional trauma of insufficient communication and sleep and sensory deprivation. Music can help shield patients—especially the comatose—from the dehumanized world they occupy on life support.[32]

When it's time to get out of bed, music can help you rehabilitate. Adding music to physical therapy for stroke victims and cerebral palsy patients increased the length and width of their steps and improved their balance.[33] Patients with chronic obstructive pulmonary disease (COPD, a lung condition that reduces breathing capacity) who exercised to music worked longer and harder—but felt it less—than patients who moved in silence.[34] Music has even been known to elicit movement in people who've been in a coma for over six months.[35]

Sara, a former trauma and critical care nurse, tells this story of how she learned about the rehabilitative power of music firsthand:

"A patient accidentally broke my neck by grabbing me and sitting on the floor—all 210 pounds of her! She died a week later, and I was a quad.

"I spent six months in the hospital and another five in a rehab facility. This Cleveland hospital had a great intern who was interested in music as therapy and used it to help me relax a bit on the ventilator. It worked, and as a result I've been using it ever since.

"It's very stressful not being able to move anything and my frustration level was reaching an all-time high. I was a black belt martial artist before my accident and very athletic. Needless to say I couldn't do that stuff anymore.

"I'm a Baroque baby at heart, so my parents got with the music therapist and we started listening to tapes of Handel, Bach, and all the other Baroque classics. I also used '50s and '60s rock and roll in rehab to keep the beat.

"After awhile, I started using music for pain control. I've had ten surgeries in as many years on my legs, ankles, back and neck—orthopedic work, which is very painful. I used a lot of biofeedback and visualization to help muscle groups work again. Yanni, Handel's Water Music . . . it sort of set the tone, if you will, for relaxation."

Even as an experienced health care professional, Sara needed help to relax under uncomfortable treatments, manage her pain, and rehabilitate. It wasn't until she became one of the patients she used to treat that she fully understood the healing qualities of music.

Braintuning Basics: Illness and Injury

Chicken Soup for the Ears

You've poured it on your soul, now try it in your ears (the author does not recommend literal interpretation). When you save certain music for curing, it can act just like chicken soup to nurture you and create the expectation of recovery. It might also bolster the production of antibodies, as certain substances in chicken soup have recently been discovered to do.

- Create your own ritual cure with music by choosing some personal favorites that make you feel relaxed, comforted, and positive. Test them with the music-mood quiz in this chapter to make sure they have a wellness effect.

- Set these CDs or tapes aside, and don't listen to them in healthy, everyday life.

- When you're sick or injured, listen to your Healing music, knowing that you chose it to make yourself well. Let it slide into your ears and down your spine like a delicious sip of soup, warming you up if you're cold or cooling you off if you're hot. Think of it as the big pot of soup your mom would make if only she were here—and just like her tender care, let the music feed your immune system and make you feel better.

Respiratory Ailments

Try music to treat lung trouble like bronchitis, asthma, or emphysema:

- Use music to structure deep breathing or accompany therapeutic coughing. Try five minute sessions, several times a day.

- Singing along to your favorite songs can also expand your lung capacity. Take half an hour a day with vocal recordings that inspire and challenge you: pop divas, Broadway musicals, choral music, and opera.[36]

Audio First Aid

Having the right music can help you through a medical emergency by lowering your blood pressure and heart rate and alleviating anxiety—so add a Walkman and a couple of tapes to your emergency kit for first aid, natural disasters, or sudden hospital trips. Make the selections soothing, perhaps at the sixty beats per minute that keeps heart attack patients calm. If you've ever been in an emergency, you know what a difference being prepared makes. Make music part of your basic first aid.

Caring for a Comatose Patient

When a loved one loses consciousness, the distress of a medical emergency is compounded by your loss of communication. Music can help you bridge the communication gap with a comatose patient, and can stimulate the physiological healing response.

Bring in some of the patient's favorite music and play it with a portable tape or CD player. Your message of care and comfort may well be perceived by the patient's mind or directly received by the body.

A Musical MRI

The technology of magnetic resonance imaging is amazing: magnetic waves actually see what's happening inside of your body, enabling doctors to diagnose otherwise invisible conditions.

Think of music as an MRI that's not just diagnostic, but healing. Hear the sound as magnetic resonance scanning your entire body. Let the frequencies balance the energy throughout your organism: your heart, lungs, nervous system, muscles, organs, cells, your mind, thoughts, and feelings. Feel it scan your invisible workings until you feel connection and flow between all the parts of your being that need to cooperate to make you well.

Back on Your Feet

The inactivity of illness is a major barrier to recovery. When you're bedridden, your muscles atrophy, your metabolism slows, and your nervous system loses power. In such a state of torpor, it's hard to even know when the disease has left your body.

When you start to feel better, let music help get you back on your feet. Prepare for your first trip out of bed by listening to some Energizing music (see Chapter 1), which will stimulate your nervous system and send electricity to your muscles before you even start to move. Let it warm you up completely before you try anything drastic.

Once you're up, try moving in time to the music. Entraining your muscles to the rhythm tunes up your coordination and helps with the ambulatory skills lost in bed. Continue with this program as necessary . . . until it takes you back to the gym.

Pain

If you're averse to illness, injury, tests, doctors, dentists, or any aspect of the medical experience, chances are that pain is the number-one reason why. In general, health care hurts—and pain itself can cause physical stress and slow your recovery. Fortunately, one of music's most extensively documented medical uses is as an audioanalgesic. It's like taking aspirin through your ears.

It's nature's intention that your body react to pain with symptoms of high stress: Increased heart rate and blood pressure. Quick, shallow breathing. Sweaty palms, knotted muscles. Sympathetic nervous system arousal and release of stress hormones. Anxiety. Even newborn babies register these responses when subjected to invasive procedures like circumcision and taking blood.

Unfortunately, these physiological responses can in turn increase your perceived level of pain, even if the pain stimulus remains constant.[37] So when pain stresses you out, that "slight pressure" the nurse has promised can feel like someone's gouging out your insides with a grapefruit spoon.

In ancient Greece, they accompanied the flogging of Ertrurian slaves with flute music to make the punishment more humane, and this trick works equally well at the dentist or during a prostate exam. Healing music can intervene in the intensifying loop between physiological and psychological distress in several ways. It relaxes your body, allowing your physical stress symptoms to diminish and lessening your experience of pain. Psychologically, music eases anxiety, which raises the threshold of what you can endure. Musical sound is a powerful distraction, taking your mind off the piece of skin that needle is about to pierce and simply letting it happen while you float with a violin or groove to a chorus. And when you choose your own pain-fighting music, you take control over an impersonal, threatening environment.

Music also acts as a mask for the unpleasant sounds that accompany many medical events, especially when played through headphones. Wouldn't you rather hear a beautiful voice than a dentist's drill? And all the cortical activity required to process music sound might even neurologically suppress the feeling of pain.[38]

The net effect is that music can both raise your pain threshold—the level of stimulus at which you first start to hurt—and decrease the ratio of your response to the intensity of the stimulus. To clarify this, consider a lab experiment that measured subjects' response to electrical shocks. People listening to vocal music endured more intense shocks before rating them uncomfortable than those who got zapped in silence. And once they crossed the pain threshold, the music listeners' responses as a function of the shocks' intensity were lower than for the silent sufferers.[39]

Audioanalgesia: How Music Relieves Pain

Healing music eases pain by acting as a:

- **Relaxant.** By lowering blood pressure, slowing pulse, loosening muscles, and deepening breathing, music can lessen your perception of pain.

- **Anxiolytic.** Music relieves anxiety, a large component of pain.

- **Distracter.** Music literally takes your mind off the pain by providing another point of focus. Listening to music of your choice also restores your sense of control.

- **Suppressor.** Some researchers believe that music might work in the brain to neurologically suppress the sensation of pain.

- **Audio screen.** Music through headphones masks the disturbing sound of procedures—drills, scraping, punching, and so forth—thus removing a source of conditioned anxiety.

One of the most successful applications of audioanalgesia has been in easing dental pain. The first study of music in the chair, published in 1948, reported that music reduced "struggling and delirium," lessened the incidence of vomiting, enabled faster emergence from anesthesia, and reduced total chair time.[40] Since then, numerous clinical studies have confirmed music's beneficial role in dental settings. Lower stress signals, less perceived pain, and decreased need for other painkillers are all good reasons to take a Walkman with you.[41] Incidentally, music you like has the most powerful painkilling effect, so don't settle for office Muzak if it's not to your taste— especially since its soothing sounds might not be as effective as loud, stimulating music for killing dental pain.

Music also scores high for alleviating pain and anxiety during invasive procedures. Its analgesic properties have proven effective during stitches, bronchoscopy, anthroscopic surgery, radiotherapy, MRIs, and flexible sigmoidoscopy, a nether-regions event so trying that patient anxiety frequently complicates or aborts the procedure.[42]

Many women welcome music in the gynecologist's office. One study that tracked patients undergoing cervical procedures including colposcopy (a microscopic examination), punch biopsy (removal of cervical tissue with a punching tool, reportedly as painful as it sounds), and cryosurgery (removal of tissue by freezing) found that music lowered pain ratings along with pulse, respiratory rate, and anxiety reports for all three procedures, with a significant reduction in overt pain for the punch biopsy. The music group undergoing biopsy also had fewer cases of excessive bleeding, which can be caused by stress symptoms that music might prevent with its relaxing effect.[43]

Another colposcopy trial with teenage girls found that watching music videos during the procedure reduced pain-related body movements and the patients' need for reassurance.[44] Music through headphones worked better than the anesthetic Methoxylflurane to relax and relieve pain in abortion patients, partly because it blocked the sound of the procedure, which the drug alone didn't do.[45] A large-scale study of 500 women found that music reduced pain during suction curettage abortions.[46]

The medical community is increasingly attuned to the devastating effects of chronic pain, which can result from injuries and diseases like rheumatoid arthritis and cancer. Regular music listening has been shown to be an effective element of chronic pain management, from structured rehabilitation programs to individual sessions for short-term relief. In one study, cancer patients "took" music two times a day along with their regularly scheduled analgesics and scored significantly lower on pain assessments than they had with medication alone. Several other studies support the effectiveness of music in treating cancer pain. Music can also increase the frequency and duration of exercise during physical therapy and results in more positive statements by chronic pain patients.[47]

Scoring a ten on the pain scale are major burns, and 75 *percent* of burn patients find that analgesics alone fail to relieve their pain. In addition to alleviating pain, music humanizes the sterile environments that burn victims must live in to guard against infection. It can also distract from routine painful treatments such as hydrotherapy, intravenous fluid therapy, joint movement, respiratory exercises, and skin grafts. For instance, playing peaceful music videos during burn dressing changes significantly reduced patients' pain intensity, pain rating indices, and anxiety. And music has been shown to help burn victims cope with grieving and trauma.[48]

Pain is a private and all-absorbing experience. Healing music can provide relief, keep you company, and pleasantly occupy your mind.

Braintuning Basics: Pain

Maximum-Strength Audioanalgesia

Here's a prescription for maximum pain relief from music:[49]

- **Use music you *like*.** Preferred music is most effective against pain and anxiety, so don't fall for the fallacy of Muzak, which might calm you down slightly but is just a placebo compared to the powerful medicine of the music you choose. And don't underestimate the positive effect of control, an added bonus that comes from making your own choice.

- **Begin the music *before* the occurrence of the pain-inducing stimulus.** Being relaxed from the start will prevent the increased pain caused by physical stress.

- **Use headphones** or, if it's available, a special pillow equipped with a speaker inside. Blocking out sound and staying in the safety of your own audio world help to distance you from distasteful events.

- **Learn to associate your pain-fighting music with pain reduction.** Try listening to the music at home first while repeating spoken affirmations such as, "I feel calm and in control." "I'm OK." "This is fine." "When I hear this music I feel all right," and so forth. Once you find music that works, use it again next time.

- **Sedate or stimulate yourself—whichever works.** In general, Relaxing music does the best job of easing the physical stress that can aggravate pain, but stimulating music has been shown to actually raise the threshold of pain at the *tactile* (nervous system), not just the perceived (mental) level, which is good for transitory and localized distress.[50] Vigorous music can also be a more powerful distracter than calmer sounds, so you might experiment with something like rock and roll to drown out the dentist's drill or divert your attention from the needle. Check the discography in chapter 1, Energize—and don't use this music for your other healing needs.

Take Two Tunes and Call Me in the Morning

Many pain sufferers have successfully used Healing music like aspirin—take it when it hurts.

- For temporary or unexpected pain, try a focused listening session when you feel the first twinge—or before, if you can anticipate it.

- If you suffer from chronic pain, schedule half an hour of focused listening into your day, two times a day or more.[51] Just as you medicate regularly (though perhaps you can give that up if you find the right music), you need regular doses of audioanalgesia to manage ongoing pain.

Rehab

If pain is coming between you and your physical therapy, use music to help you work harder and longer with less discomfort. Listening to music while you move weak or injured body parts can distract, relax, and motivate you; increase electrical activity in your muscles; and regularize gait and movement. Try a half to one hour of music and movement per day or as prescribed by your therapist.[52]

Surgery

When you're going under the knife, music can make the cut less traumatic. Listening to music before, during, and after surgery can reduce your anxiety and have you asking for less medication. It can slow the release of stress hormones into your bloodstream and lessen your chance of throwing up or having an asthma attack. And musical treatment makes it less likely that you'll experience post-traumatic stress after what is certainly a very distressing experience.

The anxiety involved in facing surgery is dramatically revealed by an experiment that measured the stress effect of simply telling patients details about surgery scheduled to be performed the next day. On average, hearing about their surgeries caused the levels of cortisol (a stress hormone) in patients' saliva to increase by 50 percent within fifteen minutes—a substantial jump indicating the trauma evoked just by thinking about their operations. Afterward, half the patients listened to music of their choice for an hour, which brought their cortisol levels back down to normal. The remaining nonmusic patients didn't recover nearly so quickly. An hour after the stressful news, their cortisol levels remained significantly higher than before.[53]

Perioperative nurses, who prepare patients for surgery, have found that music helps send people into the operating room in a calm, composed state conducive to a favorable outcome. Experiments show that preoperative music reduces fear and anxiety, gives patients a sense of control as they prepare to submit to the knife, and improves people's perceptions of the experience.[54]

The need for stress relief only increases during the operation itself, especially if you're under local or regional (as opposed to general) anesthesia. One assessment of patients who'd had surgery under nongeneral anesthesia concluded that music eased anxiety, acted as a distracter, and increased their threshold of pain,[55] while another found that it normalized patients' heart rates.[56] And a Taiwanese study that tested 120 patients undergoing epidural (spinal cord) anesthesia for surgery in both music and nonmusic conditions found that the music patients were less anxious, had lower heart rates and blood pressure, and required significantly less anesthesia.[57]

But don't think you don't need music just because the anesthesiologist has agreed to put you under. Patients under general anesthesia can perceive and remember many aspects of their operations, including disturbing sounds and words. Blocking O/R sounds with music over headphones can reduce your risk of developing post-traumatic stress disorder from memories of your surgery.[58]

Music might reduce the chance of complications, too. A team performing an abdominal operation on a severely asthmatic patient feared that the trauma of surgery might bring on an asthma attack—a dangerous situation in the middle of an operation. They added music to their anesthesia and completed the surgery smoothly.[59]

Even when they roll you into recovery, your work isn't done yet. The period following surgery can be painful and uncomfortable, and here, music's analgesic and mood-boosting powers are welcome. Especially during the first forty-eight hours of postoperative recovery, music has been shown to reduce the pain of this major trauma to your body,[60] giving you a jump start on recovery.

Postoperative gynecological and obstetric patients who listened to two hours of music a day for the two days following surgery took fewer medications and registered lower blood pressure and pulse than the nonmusic group.[61] Of sixty patients coming out of thyroid, parathyroid, or breast surgery, those who listened to music through headphones in the postanesthesia care unit waited significantly longer before requesting pain medication and reported their experience in the unit as more pleasant, both one day and one month later.[62] Researchers used half-hour music listening sessions with coronary artery bypass grafting patients in the second and third days after surgery to achieve a significant improvement in mood—an important element of recovery.[63] When patients listened to music relaxation tapes in the two days following abdominal surgery, 89 percent of them experienced less pain and distress.[64]

From beginning to end, Healing music is an effective surgical medication that's easy on your vulnerable body and good for your worried mind. Don't check in without it.

Braintuning Basics: Surgery

- Reduce preoperative anxiety and medication requirements with one-half to one hour of Healing music immediately before your surgery is scheduled.

- For a sense of calm and comfort, listen to your favorite music through headphones on the trip to the operating room.

- If possible, make arrangements with your surgeon and anesthesiologist to listen to music during surgery to disguise the ominous noises of the operating room—especially important if you're under local anesthetic.

- One-half to one and a half hours of music in postoperative recovery can help wake you up and relieve pain.

- Continue to treat yourself with music for forty-eight hours after surgery to reduce your medication needs and minimize side effects of anesthesia such as vomiting, headaches, and restlessness.[65]

Maternity

Giving birth is an exercise in rhythm, so it's no surprise that music makes it easier, from preparation to labor to delivery. Studies of obstetric patients have shown that music reduces pain, drug use, and length of labor. It improves the attitude of everyone involved, from the mother to the medical staff. Best of all, music has been found to enhance the euphoria of having a baby, helping to remind mothers that for all the hard work, this is one of the greatest pleasures in the world.

While evidence of music's ability to reduce pain and drug use in childbirth surfaced during the 1960s and '70s, the first systematic study pairing music with training, labor, and delivery was published in 1981.[66] Pregnant women in their third trimester participated in Lamaze sessions that matched music to four different levels of breathing, then listened to the music throughout labor and delivery. These mothers had significantly higher success rates on five of seven measures than the control group, including pain and discomfort, anxiety, length of labor, helpfulness of Lamaze training, and support from mates and medical staff. The researchers concluded that music worked on several levels to enhance the experience of labor and delivery, including:

- **Structured aid to breathing.** Music's rhythm and tempo provide external cues to keep you breathing regularly and deeply.

- **Focus.** Concentrating on sensory data in the music you hear helps you gain cognitive control of your pain.

- **Distraction from discomfort and pain.** The experimenters noted that a degree of intrusiveness is required in the music to successfully distract you; extremely relaxing background music doesn't qualify.

- **Conditioned relaxation.** Music you've practiced deep breathing to during training will trigger the relaxation response, allowing oxygen to flow to vital areas and keeping you calm.

- **Stimulus for pleasure response.** By setting a positive emotional tone, music reinforces the joyful aspects of giving birth.

Since this experiment was conducted, music's value during pregnancy and childbirth has been confirmed by many more studies and health care practitioners.[67]

Braintuning Basics: Maternity

- Use music during Lamaze sessions and home practice to structure your breathing and focus your attention. Concentrating on the details of the music now can help trigger your memory during childbirth.

- Add music to your prenatal exercise routine. It can regularize your movements and breathing—essential when you're pregnant.

- To help make your breathing and muscular tasks automatic and to reduce pain during labor and delivery, listen to the same music you trained to. Be prepared with several tapes so minimal deejaying is required. Remember to incorporate involving music to help distract you, and keep the tone positive to maximize euphoria (browse the discographies in this chapter and in chapter 5, Uplift).

- Consider having a special "welcome to the world" song on hand to celebrate the new arrival and reward yourself for a job well done.

- Add music to your postpartum exercise routine to inspire your efforts and ease the pain of activating those loose abdominal muscles.[68]

A Lamaze and Birthing Soundtrack

Relaxation (before Lamaze class): Slow and soft (see the discography in this chapter or in chapter 2, Relax).

Labor

- Stage I, phase I, slow chest breathing: slow, with no discernible beat. Imagine yourself floating on the sound (example: Hildegard von Bingen, *Canticles of Ecstasy* from chapter 2, Relax).

- Stage I, phase II, shallow chest or accelerated breathing: moderate-fast, increasing in speed and volume with breathing (example: Mickey Hart's *Music to Be Born By*).

- Stage I, transition, pant-blow breathing (1:1 or 4:1): faster; regulate volume to mother's wishes (example: Vivaldi's *Four Seasons*).

- Stage II, push breathing: loud; strong rhythms and distinct beat; driving melody; moderate speed (example: your favorite rock, pop, reggae or soul).

Postpartum Depression

You never expect it to happen to you, but many women come down with the blues after delivering a baby. Postpartum depression can be serious for some mothers, impairing their ability to care for the infant and in some cases leading to emotional disturbances in the new baby or other children.[69]

If you're feeling down after childbirth, refer to chapter 5, Uplift, to find out how you can use music to alleviate depression. Always seek help if your feelings are extended or severe.

Sick Children

Kids face special challenges when they're sick, especially when the illness is serious enough to require hospitalization or intrusive procedures. Uncertain about what's happening and why, emotionally immature, and dependent upon adults for satisfaction of their basic needs, hospitalized children often become fearful and depressed, which only worries parents more. Some children respond to the trauma of illness and hospitalization by withdrawing or becoming hyperactive, aggressive, or hostile, which can impede treatment and postpone the recovery process. Pediatric specialists in many areas have called for therapies to help children adjust to medical settings, so that they can get on with the important business of healing.[70] Music has proved able to answer this need.

Because it works at a nonverbal level and bypasses the need for cognitive understanding, music can reassure and stabilize even premature infants in distress. An experiment in a neonatal intensive care unit found that playing lullabies three times a day reduced the length of the infants' hospital stay by an average of five days. It also increased the babies' formula intake and daily weight gain, and decreased their stress behaviors.[71] For ventilated infants, a listening program of female vocals mixed with intrauterine sounds improved oxygen blood levels and weight gain.[72] Another study examined music's effect on preterm infants with a lung condition called bronchopulmonary dysplasia when played during suctioning—a very traumatic procedure. All the babies experienced less physiological arousal (as measured by heart rate, other autonomic indicators, and stressful facial expressions) and spent more time sleeping when surrounded by music rather than silence. Three out of four spent more time in a quiet, alert state and increased the oxygen saturation level of their blood.[73]

Because premature infants undergo many such stressful procedures at a time when they are still meant to be growing in the calm of the womb, a physiological slowdown like Healing music can be an important adjunct to medical care. The noise of neonatal ICUs can also be stressful to newborns. Like children and adults, infants have been shown to prefer music to noise, so the sound-masking effect of music can improve their environment for growth.[74]

Further evidence supports the value of music in caring for newborns,[75] but researchers have also noted that too much sensory input at critical times can harm low birth weight babies, and music interventions need to be thoroughly tested and carefully implemented.[76]

With older children, music listening and activities have been shown to reduce pain, fear, distress, and anxiety for everything from shots to terminal illness.[77] When 200 four- to six-year-olds received routine immunizations, those who heard music as the needle went in scored significantly lower on pain scales than those who didn't.[78] Pediatric burn patients had a less stressful surgery experience with music. Those who listened to relaxing music (seventy-two beats per minute or slower) before surgery with a boombox in their rooms, on the way to the O/R on Walkmans, during anesthesia induction, and in the recovery room scored significantly lower on state anxiety scales and found the whole experience more tolerable.[79]

Music is also an important nonpharmacological treatment for children with cancer. Hospitalized young cancer patients had higher levels of immunoglobin A, an immunity indicator, after listening to thirty minutes of music.[80] Music has been shown to reduce the intensity or duration of pain and the need for painkillers among child cancer patients, and to alleviate anxiety, fear, stress, and grief, even when complicated explanations don't work. Music listening activities can increase interaction, verbalization, independence, and cooperation to help the child to adjust and heal. Music facilitates exercise and physical therapy, and has even been proposed as a physiological block to the nausea center in the brain to alleviate vomiting in children undergoing chemotherapy or anesthesia.[81]

A sick child can seem heartbreakingly vulnerable, and most parents understandably agonize when they have to relinquish their children's care to others. Music provides a proactive treatment you can help design and implement for your child to provide ongoing reassurance—even when you're not there.

Braintuning Basics: Sick Children

Newborns

Babies learn to distinguish their mother's voice within two hours of birth, and it's been shown that the most effective lullaby for calming a newborn baby is that voice, so if you're able, start singing as soon as you can.

But taped music can be an effective treatment when mom isn't available, especially for premature and low birth weight infants who must remain in the neonate unit until they've grown enough to go home. If you're the parent of a hospitalized newborn:

- Find out what your hospital's policy is on music, noise, and other stimulus.

- If the neonate unit does play music, it should be very soothing, at a level of about seventy to eighty decibels, and keyed to the baby's daily rhythms. Infants prefer vocal to instrumental music, and music in the heartbeat range of sixty to eighty beats per minute may be the most comforting.

- If the hospital doesn't play music to neonates, see if you can make your own arrangements. Enlist a unit nurse you trust to implement your plan. Make a tape of yourself singing lullabies at a relaxed, steady tempo to stay in touch with your hospitalized baby.

Make a Plan

When your child is hospitalized, remember that the nursing staff holds the key to the young patient's daily care. If you would like music played in your absence, provide the equipment and recordings and consult with the nurse about appropriate selections and timing. Most nurses are happy to have additional tools at their disposal, and many will be experienced in using music therapy to care for children.

At Home

Make music part of your treatment when you care for a sick child at home. Try Healing music:

- When your child fusses or complains of pain

- To facilitate feeding, bathing, administering medicine, or other difficult procedures

You can also use your child's favorite music (it need not have healing characteristics) as a reward for good behaviors like taking medicine, and to encourage play and communication.

Aging, Death, and Dying

Nancy said, "My father went into a nursing home two months ago, and when I visit him, he asks me to sing. I do (softly so as not to bother other residents), and I believe that it's therapeutic for him for two reasons: because it's music and because it's his daughter."

For Nancy, singing provides a way of caring for her father as he makes a difficult transition into full-time and permanent health care. When medical treatment becomes a long-term proposition, music can humanize the experience and help at both physical and emotional levels. These include pain control, communication, and quality of life.

One use of music with elderly patients is to manage behavior when cognitive processes start to slip. For instance, playing music in a nursing home dining hall has been shown to reduce the agitated behaviors of residents with cognitive impairment.[82] Music has also been widely used with Alzheimer's patients, to facilitate communication, spur happy memories, and reduce disruptive exclamations.[83] Music therapy can also help both the patient and loved ones cope with the mourning and grief caused by the sudden mental and physical impairments of neurological disease.[84]

Music's well-documented power over pain is welcomed by many terminal patients who live with the knowledge that they will never witness complete relief. Many medical professionals are now concerned about the rise of addiction to painkillers and tranquilizers among the elderly, caused by the hardships of facing illness, pain, loneliness, and the end of life.[85] When mind and body start to lose their power, Healing music can provide nonpharmacological relief and comfort. Music can also relieve fear and anxiety about death, relieve depression, and facilitate the grieving process in facing the end of life.[86]

Recent growth in the field of death education reflects people's increasing concern over quality of life for the dying. Knowledge and a conscious approach to the last days of life can make them more rewarding and comfortable for both the patient and loved ones. The emerging field of music-thanatology uses music to attend to the physical and spiritual needs of people approaching death. Tracing its historical roots back to French monastic medicine, in which "infirmary music" was used toward the goal of conscious dying and blessed death, music-thanatology today is becoming a valued practice for patients with terminal cancer, AIDS, and degenerative disease. Playing Healing music in bedside vigils in homes, hospitals, and hospices provides a way to mark and share the passage from life.[87]

Braintuning Basics: Aging, Death, and Dying

Use the techniques for pain control and healing throughout this chapter to ease the traumas of aging and terminal illness. If you're caring for a terminal patient, remember the power of Healing music to control pain and enhance quality of life. Find out about the patient's music preferences and make well-loved selections part of your treatment plan.

The Heal Music-Mood Checklist

❑ Personal preference

❑ Steady, flowing pulse

❑ Slow to moderate tempo (sixty to eighty beats per minute)

❑ Moderate, constant volume

❑ Human voice (especially for infants)

❑ Strings and other soothing tone colors

❑ Familiarity

❑ For brief pain: Energizing music (see chapter 1)

Avoid stimulating music if you're anxious, stressed, or traumatized. See the section on maternity for music recommended for labor and childbirth.[88] See also chapter 2, Relax, for many more selections that share healing characteristics.

Test Your Musical Dosage

See page 24 in the introduction for instructions on testing your music-mood response. A Heal discography follows the quiz. Start by testing your favorite styles from the list and recording your results in the journal that follows. Note that this quiz is slightly different than those in other chapters, measuring your feelings on a qualitative scale.

The Heal Music-Mood Test

Rate yourself in each spectrum below, giving the word on the left a value of 1 and the word on the right a value of 5. Repeat after listening.

	Before Listening	After Listening	Change, Before to After
I Feel	(1–5)	(1–5)	(+ or –, 0–4)
Tense—Relaxed	_____	_____	_____
Weak—Strong	_____	_____	_____
Vulnerable—Safe	_____	_____	_____
Hurting—Relieved	_____	_____	_____
Queasy—Calm	_____	_____	_____
Injured—Healed	_____	_____	_____
Distressed—Soothed	_____	_____	_____
Broken—Mended	_____	_____	_____
Worried—Reassured	_____	_____	_____
Sick—Well	_____	_____	_____

Total Change:
Your Musical Dosage (0–40) _____

The Heal Music-Mood Journal

Date	Situation	Selection	Score
_____	_____	_____	_____
_____	_____	_____	_____
_____	_____	_____	_____
_____	_____	_____	_____
_____	_____	_____	_____
_____	_____	_____	_____
_____	_____	_____	_____
_____	_____	_____	_____
_____	_____	_____	_____
_____	_____	_____	_____
_____	_____	_____	_____
_____	_____	_____	_____
_____	_____	_____	_____
_____	_____	_____	_____
_____	_____	_____	_____
_____	_____	_____	_____
_____	_____	_____	_____
_____	_____	_____	_____
_____	_____	_____	_____
_____	_____	_____	_____

Braintuning Music: Heal

As early as 1929, researchers determined that music's effect on patients' blood pressure was determined less by the musical style than by the patient's appreciation of it. Because noise can interfere with your recovery and music can enhance it, the first criteria for choosing music to heal by is that you like it very much—perceiving it as delightful, not as annoying noise. That means that if you're sick or healing, you should refuse exposure to music you don't like, and instead surround yourself with sounds that make you feel good.

While the suggestions below and cross-references to other chapters give you guidelines and many options to explore, the best healing music is what *you* choose.

Vocal Music

Many people retain the strong emotional connection to the human voice evidenced by newborn babies, and the predominance of vocals in healing music around the world suggests global agreement on the issue. In addition to the primacy of its emotional impact, vocal music can help take your mind off the pain with words. Uplifting lyrics, as in sacred songs or some styles of pop, provide hope and comfort.

But beware—there's plenty of negative vocal music out there. Avoid angst and doubt in the songs you listen to during this vulnerable time.

Familiar Classics

People report feeling better to familiar classical pieces like Vivaldi's *Four Seasons* or Debussy's *Prelude to the Afternoon of the Faun* when they're sick. Any classical selection that makes you feel relaxed and comfortable is a good choice for healing. The discography includes many of these, as well as some you might not know yet but whose warmth and rich imagery can help lift you out of your current state of mind and body. Is there a piece or composer that reliably comforts and assures you? Add it to your list.

Harps

Harps have been used for healing since the ancient Greeks and have shown up as cures in Biblical scripture and secular literature.[89] Choose from Celtic harps, medieval versions, the West African *kora* (harp-lute), the many South American variations adopted after the Spanish invasion, or the angelic sound of the Western concert harp.

Drones

Many spirit and meditative musics are grounded on the sound of a drone, or low, steady tone. Found in the Indian *tambour* that accompanies the *sitar* and other instruments, the Chinese *sho*, Australian *didgeridoo*, bagpipes, and the chanting of "om," the unceasing sound of a single tone has a special and recognizable effect. Some people believe that the drone is a healing sound that vibrates in the body to dispel blockages and touch specific sites. The *didgeridoo*, for instance, has an unmistakable bass resonance you might recognize from the Foster's beer commercials. Used by the Aborigines in a secret sacred ceremony called the *corroboree*, the instrument is a eucalyptus log hollowed out by termites and is played by blowing into the end. It's one of the most other-worldly experiences sound can provide.

While the use of drones around the world is too widespread to specifically ascribe to healing, you might find the sound works for you.

World Healing Music

Many trance and shamanic music practices have healing as their object. Native American cultures have songs to treat both specific and general ills. In Morocco, Gnawan musicians play trance music for *derdeba* healing ceremonies. The Chinese have an elaborate conception of music and medicine that involves *yin-yang* balance, the five elements of nature and the internal organs of the body.

Note that the act of recording music can separate it from the power of human healers and the original ritual context that support its beneficial effects. But the aural impact remains intact, and can have discernible physiological effects on the body. In fact, while insiders might say that their music heals by extracting the soul or calling the ancestors, an outsider might analyze how it calms the nervous system or stimulates the cortex.

Healing Music In Other Chapters

Here are some important cross-references to help you explore more music for healing:

- The selections in **chapter 2, Relax**, share the characteristics of Healing music. Turn to them to calm down, control ongoing pain, and lessen the stress that illness puts on your body and mind. Many of the trance musics described in chapter 2 are also believed to have healing properties.

- When bed rest leaves you needing a boost to your circulation, try some **Energizing or Uplifting music (chapters 1 and 5)**. When it's time, the physiological priming effect of these musical styles can actually help power you out of bed.

- **Energizing music (chapter 1)** is also helpful for short-term pain. Its stimulating qualities make the best distraction and raise your tactile pain threshold.

The Braintuning Discography: Heal

STYLE	TITLE
Vocal Music	• *Amazing Grace—A Country Salute to Gospel*. Sparrow 1445. Alison Krause, Charlie Daniels, Emmylou Harris and others perform quiet takes on gospel songs classic and new. • Crosby, Stills, Nash & Young. *So Far*. Atlantic 82648. Strong medicine for children of the '60s. • The Fairfield Four. *Standing in the Safety Zone*. Warner Brothers 26945. This a cappella gospel group was founded in the 1920s and the current line-up still delivers soaring leads and deep bass. • Aretha Franklin. *Aretha Gospel*. Chess/MCA 91521. A young Aretha wails slow, expressive hymns to bare piano and organ accompaniment and ecstatic cries from the audience. • Nusrat Fateh Ali Khan. *Devotional & Love Songs*. Real World/Virgin 2300. Vocal pyrotechnics from one of Pakistan's most revered singers of *qawwali*, or sacred songs. • Dolly Parton, Linda Ronstadt, and Emmylou Harris. *Trio*. Warner Brothers 25491. Angelic voices sing country, pop, and gospel; try the classic "Farther Along." • Take 6. *Take 6*. Reprise 25670. A cappella gospel group. • Zap Mama. *Sabsylma*. Warner Brothers 45537. Afro–European ensemble of women use their vocal chords like an orchestra, choir, and rhythm section. • SEE ALSO vocal music, including lullabies, in chapter 2, Relax.
Familiar Classics	• Johann Sebastian Bach. *6 Brandenburg Concertos BWV 1046–1051*. Trevor Pinnock, The English Concert, Archive 423492. • Ludwig van Beethoven. "Cavatina" from *String Quartet in B-flat Major, Op. 130* on *Key to the Quartets*. The Emerson String

Quartet, Deutsche Grammophon 447083. The comforting sonority and subtle, vibrating energy of strings.

• Hector Berlioz. Love Scene from *Roméo et Juliette* on *Berlioz: La Marseillaise*. David Zinman & the Baltimore Symphony Orchestra, Telarc 80164. Tender melodies and romantic imagery to take you away from your present surroundings. The 16-minute length makes a good analgesic.

• Anton Bruckner. "Ave Maria for alto and organ in F" on *The Choral Works of Anton Bruckner*. Paul Shewan Roberts & the Wesleyan College Chorale, Albany 34061–63.

• Aaron Copland. First movement of *Clarinet Concerto*. Leonard Bernstein & the New York Philharmonic, Deutsche Grammophon 431672. A meditative movement that lets the clarinet sing.

• Claude Debussy:

3 "Nocturnes" on *Daphne et Chloe Suite No. 2*. Paul Paray & the Detroit Symphony Orchestra, Mercury Living Presence 34306. Debussy's nighttime portraits for orchestra and chorus are sometimes dreamy, other times mystical, always transporting.

Prelude to the Afternoon of the Faun. Pierre Boulez & the Cleveland Orchestra, Deutsche Grammophon 435766. Sweet flute melodies and washes of harp take you to a magical place. Close your eyes and try to see the fauns gamboling about on a grassy knoll.

• Antonín Dvořák. *Nocturne for String Orchestra*. Orpheus Chamber Orchestra, Deutsche Grammophon 431680. Adds the shimmer of strings to the dark of night.

• George Frideric Handel. *3 Suites ("Water Music"), HWV 348–350*, Archive 410525.

• Gustav Holst. "Venus, the Bringer of Peace" on *The Planets*. James Levine & the Chicago Symphony Orchestra, Deutsche Grammophon 429730. Take a lyrical trip into the stratosphere with a full orchestra and healing harp to lead the way.

• Wolfgang Amadeus Mozart:

Clarinet Quintet in A Major, K. 581. David Shifrin and Chamber Music Northwest, Delos 3020. The soft, warm clarinet is one of Mozart's sweetest voices; here it joins with strings for soothing chamber music.

Kathleen Battle Sings Mozart. André Previn & the Royal Philharmonic Orchestra. EMI/Angel 47355. Tender arias in delicate renditions by a great soprano.

Arvo Part. *Tabula Rasa*. Kremer, Jarret, ECM 21275.

• Franz Schubert. "Ave Maria for voice and piano in B-flat" on *Ave Maria/Lieder*. Elly Ameling, Philips 420870. Many composers have set the Ave Maria to music; Schubert's version is the most famous.

• Richard Strauss. *Four Last Songs*. Gundula Janowitz, Herbert von Karajan & the Berlin Philharmonic, Deutsche Grammophon 447422. Soprano and orchestra in a rhapsodic union that would be worthy of the last music on earth.

• Antonio Vivaldi. *The Four Seasons*. Gil Shaham & the Orpheus Chamber Orchestra, Deutsche Grammophon 439933.

• Richard Wagner. *Siegfried-Idyll*. Orpheus Chamber Orchestra, Deutsche Grammophon 431680. Join Siegfried in his orchestral daydream of bliss.

SEE ALSO the discussion of slow or "adagio" movements in chapter 2, Relax.

Harp

• *Caprices and Fantasies: Romantic Harp Music of the 19th Century*. Susan Drake, Hyperion 66340. Includes Debussy's "Clair de Lune"; could be better than a sleeping pill.

• *Celtic Treasure: The Legacy of Turlough O'Carolan*. Narada 63925. Contemporary Celtic musicians play the compositions of 17th-century blind Irish composer Carolan. Beautiful harping with overtones of the Baroque.

• The Chieftains. *The Celtic Harp: A Tribute to Edward Bunting*. RCA Victor 61490. Some tracks include the entire Belfast Harp Orchestra.

• Vieux Diop. *Vieux Diop (Via Jo)*. Worldly/Triloka 7209. The West African *kora*, or harp-lute, presented in contemporary arrangements with lush production.

• Carlo Gesualdo. *Madrigeaux (Madrigals)*. William Christie & Les Arts Florissant Ensemble, Harmonia Mundi 901268. Delicate vocal settings by an Italian Renaissance prince include ethereal harp interludes.

• Amadu Bansang Jobarteh. *Tabara: Gambian Kora Music*. Music of the World 129. From West Africa—cascading harp lines, reassuring hums, and songs about the past, the future, and long life.

• Claudio Monteverdi. *Orfeo*. Gwendolyn Toth & Artek, Lyrichord 9002. An entire opera about the healing harp.

• *A Song for Francesca: Music in Italy, 1330–1400*. Christopher Page & the Gothic Voices, Hyperion 66286. Medieval vocal and harp music.

• *The Service of Venus and Mars—Music for Knights of Garter*. Christopher Page & the Gothic Voices, Andrew Lawrence-King. Hyperion 66238. These English and French pieces for voice and harp were favorites of the 14th-century Knights of Garter, a distinguished group of lords that included founder King Edward III as well as King Henry V.

Drones

• Kay Gardner. *Drone Zone*. The Relaxation Company 3188. This American composer plays flute over drones from around the world. While world music fans might prefer to seek out the real thing, the long tones are gentle and soothing.

• Adam Plack, Johnny (White Ant) Soames, William Brady & Luke Cummins. *Dawn Until Dusk: Tribal Song and Didgeridoo*. Australian Music International 3003. Recorded on location in the Outback, the deep, droning Australian instrument called the *didgeridoo* is accompanied by the sounds of birds, bugs, and thumping kangaroos. Several totem songs provide additional protection. (Skip vocal tracks #2, 4, 6, 9, and 11 if you strictly seek the resonance of the drone.)

• Adam Plack & Johnny (White Ant) Soames. *Winds of Warning*. Australian Music International 2002. This world music mix adds rich arrangements and instrumentation to the sound of the *digeridoo*. The results score higher on the intensity scale than many other Heal selections—but the sound really vibrates.

• Ravi Shankar & Ali Akbar Khan. *Ragas*. Fantasy 24714. A hypnotic *tambour* drone underlies four extended ragas by the sitarist whose music has been clinically proven to lower stress hormone levels, and the great *sarod* player Khan.

Native American Healing Songs

• *Between Father Sky and Mother Earth: A Native American Collection*. Narada 63915. A rare combination of mostly traditional Native music with high-quality studio production. Includes Healing songs in Sioux and Navajo.

• *Songs of Earth, Water, Fire and Sky: Music of the American Indian*. New World 80246. The Yurok Women's Brush Dance is for healing a sick child; the Navajo Ribbon Dance helps troublesome throats.

• *Songs of the Spirit*. Worldly/Triloka 4137. This Native American compilation mixes traditional music, including a Creek medicine flute, with haunting studio production.

• Cornel Pewardy & the Alliance West Singers. "Kiowa Hymns" I, II, and III, "Love Song," "Comanche Flute Solo," and "Land of Enchantment" on *Dancing Buffalo*. Music of the World-130. Unaccompanied vocal hymns and solo pieces on the beautiful Kiowa flute.

Chinese Healing Music

• Central Chinese Music College Orchestra. *Five Tones Healing Music—Kung, Shang, Chueh, Jyy, Yu, and Regimen-Qi Circulation*. Wind 3115–3120. The 5 tones of Chinese music are said to correspond to 5 organs or systems in the body, and this 6-CD set explores each one.

• Shanghai Chinese Traditional Orchestra. *Yi-Ching Music for Health—Metal, Wood, Water, Fire, Earth, and Regimen*. Wind

3109-3114. 5 CDs based on *yin–yang* theory, with each element corresponding to specific healing applications.

    • Shanghai Chinese Traditional Orchestra. *Chinese Medical Psychosomatic Music Therapy.* Wind. Also based on *yin*, *yang*, and the 5 elements, each of these discs focuses on a particular ailment: Hypertension (3123), Intestinal Ulceration (3124), Headache (3125), Dysmenorrhea (3126), Constipation (3127), Climacteric Syndrome (3128), Obesity (3129), Cancer (3130), Stroke (3131), and Coronary Arteriosclerosis (3132).

Malaysian Dream-songs	• *Dream Songs and Healing Sounds in the Rainforests of Malaysia.* Recorded, compiled, and annotated by Marina Roseman, Folkways/ Smithsonian 40417. Songs and trance dances from the Temiar people.
Moroccan Gnawa	• Hassan Hakmoun. *The Fire Within: Gnawa Music of Morocco.* Music of the World 135. Son of a *shuwafa* healer, Hakmoun performs trance music on the *sintir*, or bass lute, with finger cymbal accompaniment. SEE ALSO trance music in chapter 2, Relax.

Childbirth Music	• Mickey Hart. *Music to be Born By.* Rykodisc 20112. Ambient world beat sounds based on the pre-natal heartbeat. Mothers report that the predictable 16-beat cycle is very nice—until it comes time to push.
	    • Gladys Knight & the Pips. *Imagination.* Buddah 49504. Recommended by a nurse specializing in musical childbirth.[90]
	    • Your favorite rock, pop, or soul. (See the specific recommendations for different stages of labor earlier in the chapter.)

See page 255 for Sources.

Heal: The Braintuning 5

A diverse sampling from the discography to get you started:

- Take 6. *Take 6*. Reprise 25670.

- Claude Debussy. *Prelude to the Afternoon of the Faun*. Pierre Boulez & the Cleveland Orchestra, Deutsche Grammophon 435766.

- *Celtic Treasure: The Legacy of Turlough O'Carolan*. Narada 63925.

- Ravi Shankar & Ali Akbar Khan. *Ragas*. Fantasy 24714.

- Hassan Hakmoun. *The Fire Within: Gnawa Music of Morocco*. Music of the World 135.

Music Is My Medicine

Just as you might not think that you're taking medicine when you eat an orange, you probably don't associate music with healing properties on a daily basis. But both the vitamins in oranges and the psychophysiological properties of music can go a long way toward making and keeping you well. When you're preventing illness, fighting pain, or healing, remember that a new view of your daily musical diet can turn it into potent and proven medicine.

Uplift

You don't need a research team to tell you that music makes you feel good. Jamming for joy is as old as music itself, and it's widely agreed that music operates at psychophysiological, emotional, aesthetic, social, cultural, and spiritual levels to help you have fun. But its mood-boosting powers can also be more specific and useful than that. The elevating music in this chapter stimulates optimism, breaks emotional paralysis, and provides a natural energy lift—an antidepressant with no side effects.

Uplift Overview

Uplifting Music Can Help You With:	Use These Techniques if You Are:	How Music Helps:
Temporary Setbacks and Sadness	Suffering from a disappointment, failure, or loss	Induces an elated mood.
Depression	Feeling down, paralyzed, hopeless, or fatigued.	Improves your mood; raises your physiological arousal to normal levels; provides an easy way to be proactive.

Negative or Recurrent Thoughts	Experiencing unwanted or intrusive thoughts; obsessing over a problem or detail.	Creates a positive outlook to clear negative cognitions from your mind; acts as distraction.
Overeating	Eating to feel better or boost your mood; occasionally or constantly obsessed with food.	Induces a better mood to help you skip food you don't need.
Shyness	Anxious about interacting with people effectively; limited by self-doubt.	Lifts your spirits and energy; creates a shared feeling of bonhomie; stimulates your system to alleviate fear of rejection.

When you think of mood, words like happiness and sadness might come to mind. Clinically, we speak of elated, depressed, and neutral moods. No matter how you term it, the latest research into biochemistry and mood indicates that where you sit on the happy-to-sad spectrum can affect how you work, relate, eat, sleep, and feel about yourself. The recent wave of interest in Prozac and other antidepressant drugs is linked to new and developing studies showing that people exhibit infinite variations on the biochemical mix that determines their mood on a daily basis—and that many people wish they felt better.

Using music to treat depression was one of the original applications of the practice of music therapy. Now, music's ability to induce *both* elated and depressed moods is clinically proven,[1] so the right listening strategy is critical to creating and maintaining a positive, productive outlook.

Music can help you feel happier on an ongoing or as-needed basis. But a musical misstep at a time of emotional vulnerability can make you feel worse, so this chapter provides the tools you need to make the right choices for your good mood.

Temporary Setbacks and Sadness

Things go wrong. And when they do, sadness or a low mood is a natural reaction. When you've lost in love, been turned down for a job, had plans fall through or a goal shot down, a plummet in your mood state is to be expected. Experience your sadness if that seems right. And then let music make you feel better again.

Marie, a habilitation training specialist, cues up the Grateful Dead when she feels down. "They transport me to a totally other place. Music can change the world." She adds her own precaution: "Nine Inch Nails and such can just depress a person more." Bill lost his job to corporate downsizing and reports spending an entire weekend with his '60s soul collection to generate the energy to work on his résumé.

The Chinese character for music also means *happy*. That quality does seem inherent to certain kinds of music, and the most common application of musical mood induction, a well-established music therapy technique, is making sad people happy. Experiments using psychological mood-rating scales and measurements of physiological arousal have proven music's ability to induce elated, depressed, and neutral moods. In fact, musical mood induction tends to have greater success and fewer gender differences than other mood arousal techniques.[2]

The first thing Uplifting music does is perk up your body, raising heart and respiratory rates and blood pressure—which tend to sink with low moods—to make you feel more alive. Concurrent with or as a result of these changes, your mood improves as measured by various standardized tests, self-assessments, or reactions to other stimulis. In fact, changing your mood with music can change the way you see the world. One study found that musical mood induction significantly altered subjects' perceptions of the expressions on people's faces.[3]

When the emotional forecast is trending down, look up with music.

Braintuning Basics: Setbacks and Sadness

Make Yourself Happy

Music you like is the least you deserve in this difficult moment, and it also seems to do the best job of picking up the pace of your vital functions.[4] You're fragile just now, so treat yourself to your Uplifting favorites, and run screaming from any music that doesn't make you happy.

Lift-Off

Use this visualization technique to boost music's mood-lifting power:

- Think of the music as a golden light filling your head. Every beat that hits your ears makes the light shine brighter, like an electrical current.

- Move the light to the top of your head, warming up your scalp from below.

- Now let the top of your head lift off and the light beam upward. Feel the circuit you create as music enters your ears, turns into energy, and shines a light straight up into the sky.

PMS Power

PMS can make you listless and lethargic—the same symptoms associated with sadness and depression. Uplifting music can help you out of your hormonal slump:

- Start with a focused listening session when the first symptoms strike. Drop what you're doing and treat yourself to ten minutes of doing nothing but listening to Uplifting music.

- Continue to surround yourself with as much Uplifting music as you can for as long as your symptoms last. Play it softly in the background while you work, or take listening breaks when you feel yourself bottoming out.

See the following section for more braintuning techniques to treat temporary sadness.

Depression

An estimated seventeen million Americans suffer from depression in any given year,[5] living with the double bind of emotional distress and decreased productivity and energy levels. The group of affective mood disorders termed depression can cloud your thinking, disrupt your emotional stability, and undermine your ability to cope with stress. Feeling bad often erodes your desire to do and achieve, which can eat away at your self-esteem and make you feel even worse. It can bring fatigue, pessimism, and poor concentration. Whether you're fighting a dark feeling when daylight saving time ends or dealing with an ongoing loss of hope and optimism, depression can kill your daily joy in being alive.

Up to 50 percent of depression cases go undiagnosed, therefore untreated. The psychological community is concerned about this shortfall because there's so much to be gained from feeling better. Treating depression can make you more cheerful, self-assured, and relaxed. Being in a better mood can help you concentrate, and so be more productive, clear, and articulate. It can stimulate your immune system. It can free you from paralysis when every course of action looks like a potential failure. Improving your emotional outlook can give you the power and energy to face what looms and threatens, and music can help get you there.

Depression: The Details

Depression is an affective disorder that can be further classified into several types. The symptoms include sadness, lack of interest in daily life, less enjoyment of pleasurable things, poor attention and concentration, low self-esteem, sleep disruption, altered appetite, and a sense of hopelessness or helplessness. Episodes of these feelings that last two weeks or more and interfere with daily activities are generally diagnosed as depression.

- Experts estimate that 5 to 20 percent of the population is clinically depressed.

- Up to 50 percent of cases of depression go undiagnosed.

- In the past, women were considered twice as likely to be depressed as men, but recent psychological findings suggest that covert depression might be more prevalent among men than previously thought, and depression could hit men as hard as women.

- Other risk factors include being unmarried or unattached, and experiencing a personal loss.[6]

They say that Philip V of Spain was cured of depression by opera arias performed by the Italian singer Farinelli.[7] This is clinically feasible, as music can be used as an on-the-spot treatment to induce an elated mood and improve self-esteem. In one study, people with both high and low self-esteem felt better about themselves after using music to attain a positive mood.[8] Music has also been successfully used as part of long-term strategies to treat both minor and major depression, decreasing scores on depression test scales and improving outlook and mood.

Just as happy music can make you feel better, listening to sad or negative music can make you feel worse. A study of music as a suicide risk factor for teenagers, for instance, associated rock and heavy metal music with depression and suicidal thoughts, and found that it made at-risk teens sadder.[9] Likewise, musical mood induction can work both ways. Melancholy music has been shown to increase depression in listeners.[10]

It seems we get sadder as we age. A study that asked people to ascribe emotions to different pieces of music found agreement across gender lines and levels of musical expertise about what music expressed which emotion, but adults overall perceived less happiness and more anger in music than children.[11] In the Netherlands, researchers found that children ascribe simple parameters of happiness and sadness to music, but adults work with a more complex hierarchy of positive and negative values that include fear.[12]

If growing up means gaining emotional range, remember music as a balancing force to help you maintain equilibrium.

You're Never Too Old or Too Young to Feel Bad

Older adults have a fairly high incidence of depression (about 10 percent of people over sixty-five), and a good deal of the research in treating depression with music has been conducted with this group. Various kinds of music therapy, including listening, have been effective in lifting depression for older adults, and might even succeed where other psychotherapeutic techniques fail.[13]

Over 90 percent of depression cases in the elderly go untreated. Limited resources or inability to leave the home might prevent older adults from seeking treatment. Fortunately, music listening has been shown to be an effective home-based intervention for depression with significant and sustainable results.

Children can also be depressed, and many teachers and caregivers are uncertain how to help. Some experts recommend treating depression in the classroom with strategies that include music.[14]

Braintuning Basics: Depression

Just Push Play

Depression has a tendency to paralyze people, making them passive, motionless, stunned. The longer you sit still, the more your nervous system slows down, sending you into a descending spiral.

Prepare yourself for bouts of depression with braintuning techniques *before* you find yourself frozen on the couch:

- Expand on a popular depression therapy and mark your favorite Uplifting CDs with the adhesive blue dots available in office supply shops. If you make your own vectoring tapes (see below), mark those with dots too. Keep your Uplifting music collection on display in plain sight so that when you start to feel down, all you have to do is scan for a blue dot.

- Keep an Uplift selection cued up in your tape or CD player and have one or more remote controls on hand so that you can start the music without getting up.

- When bad feelings hit, just push Play. Simply making the decision to treat yourself to some Uplifting music can make you feel better— and if not now, when?

Liatris, a bookstore owner who suffers from depression, offers this first-hand advice:

"You're not immobilized at the moment, or you wouldn't have the energy to read this, so go make a tape *right now* or at the very least put little blue dot stickers on the spines of the CDs that might work, because you *know* that when push comes to shove, you'd rather sit and smoke cigarettes or drink or stare at the wall."

The Elation Elevator

One of the best ways to musically boost your mood is gradually—starting at a slow or moderate pace close to the way you're feeling now and getting more uplifting with each selection. This is the iso or vectoring technique described in the Introduction as one of the most effective ways to induce mood with music. People listening to such a progression of music report feeling "relaxed but excited, with increased energy and spirit."[15]

To take advantage of vectored mood induction, make your own graduated elation tape:

- Start with slow or midtempo music that matches the way you tend to feel when you're depressed.

- Make each selection increasingly faster, more upbeat, and higher in pitch. Go *gradually*. Pushing your mood too fast might make you anxious or resentful.

- Limit the total time to what you might reasonably listen to in a down moment, and make the last number your personal expression of hallelujah.

- Make one or more elevation tapes, mark them with blue dots, and keep them close at hand. When you need a boost, follow the instructions for Just Push Play on page 167.

The Iso Uplift: Two Variations

Following are two different examples of sequences for gradually lifting your mood using the iso principle and selections from the discography. Whether you prefer the jazz/soul/funk/rock series or the classical pieces, either sequence should have you feeling better in fifteen to twenty minutes—or use the examples as a basis for making longer tapes.

JAZZ/SOUL/FUNK/ROCK

1. Nat King Cole Trio, "Sweet Lorraine" (*Esquire—The Voice of the Soul*, from chapter 2, Relax). A sweet jazz tune at the upper end of the heartbeat range (90 beats per minute) with hopeful lyrics and simple instrumentation. Relaxing selections make a good, low-key start when you're using the iso principle.
2. The Staple Singers, "I'll Take You There" (*Top of the Stax: Twenty Greatest Hits*). This classic soul tune takes the tempo up to 104 beats per minute and adds fuller instrumentation and gospel-tinged vocals with an answering chorus.
3. Sly & the Family Stone, "You Can Make It If You Try" (*Greatest Hits*). The tempo remains the same (104), but the funky groove, hard-hitting horns, and emphatically encouraging lyrics all add to the intensity.
4. The Eagles, "Take It Easy" (*Their Greatest Hits*). The loose rhythmic feel of this well-loved rock song makes the jump up to 138 beats per minute easy. With

music and a message that are both encouraging and destressing, you should finish feeling hopeful and free.

CLASSICAL

1. Nicolo Paganini, "Rondo" from *Sonata Concertata M.S. 2* (*Paganini for Two*). This duet for violin and guitar moves at 112 beats per minute in a lilting triple meter. The friendly dialogue between instruments will have you tapping your toe; the simple texture is an undemanding way to begin your listening.
2. Adrian LeRoy, "Une m'avoit promis" (*La Roque 'n' Roll*). An upbeat *chanson* from Renaissance France, this selection keeps the swing of the previous one, speeds the tempo to 120 beats per minute, and adds sprightly vocal and flute lines.
3. W. A. Mozart, "Rondo" from *Eine Kleine Nachtmusik*. Though still moving at 120 beats per minute, this piece's bouncy theme gives the impression of much more rhythmic action, with a full string orchestra to add to the effect.
4. Gustav Holst, "Jupiter, the Bringer of Jollity" from *The Planets*. This grand orchestral piece is like a liberating trip into the solar system. With majestic horn fanfares, broad, sweet themes, and thundering timpani, it should have the firepower to drive away any lingering fog.

Sometimes you'll discover the iso principle within a single song—like "Try a Little Tenderness" by Otis Redding or "Free Bird" by Lynyrd Skynyrd. Songs that start slow and gradually build in intensity and speed are mini-uplift sequences; give them a try when time is short or you don't want to deal with a tape or swapping CDs.

Depression and Anxiety

For some people, depression comes accompanied by anxiety, the state of physiological and emotional vigilance described in chapter 2, Relax. If you listen to the upbeat music featured in this chapter in an anxious mood, it might make you nervous or annoyed instead of elated.

If you're feeling depressed and anxious, ease into your braintuning treatment:

- Start with music from chapter 2, Relax. Unwind until the music takes the edge off your anxiety.

- Continue with a gentle vectoring program as described above, very gradually working your way up the arousal scale. If you feel your anxiety return, stop and return to music and techniques from chapter 2. Chances are that the time isn't right for you to self-stimulate with music.

Lyrics: A Cognitive Boost

Some experiments in musical mood induction have found that music's effect is significantly enhanced by adding positive verbal messages—taking the process beyond the affective realm and into the cognitive.[16]

Homo sapiens must have instinctually known about the link between verbal cognition and mood when they first started singing songs with lyrics. To take your mood induction the final mile, choose songs with positive, inspiring lyrics to reinforce the music's uplifting message.

Get Rhythm

Evidence suggests that depressed people exhibit decreased rhythmic competence, and that their timekeeping abilities actually improve as antidepressant medication kicks in and mood improves.[17]

You can extrapolate this finding to propose that getting rhythm beats the blues. So reinforce your alignment with time by clapping and moving to music for a little locomotion therapy—and a restart for your system.

Happy Days

Many people get a mood boost from music they associate with happy times in the past. A six-month observation of elderly patients who listened to 1920s and '30s big band jazz—music of their youth that also happens to meet Uplifting criteria—found them happier, more alert, and better able to recall their personal histories than two control groups who did puzzles or drew pictures.[18]

Music is a potent reminder of past moments and their emotional contexts, and playing music that you remember from a time of success, excitement, or happiness can help return you to that state.[19]

Listen with Your Inner Child's Ear

It's proven that children perceive more happiness in music than grown-ups,[20] so when you're listening for an uplifting effect, try to experience the music as a child would. Delight in its rhythms and surprises. Picture the last time you saw a toddler spontaneously dance to music. Now put yourself in her ears.

You might try changing your mood with a childhood favorite like "Peter and the Wolf" or "Jungle Book"—or sneak in some innocent fun by playing Christmas carols in July.

Negative or Recurrent Thoughts

Lisa lived through the Northridge earthquake of 1994 and for the next two years was tormented by flashbacks and uninvited thoughts about the quake, which interfered with her work and sleep. It seemed like the thoughts were self-spawning: whenever one worked its way into her mind, many more followed. The only way Lisa could clear her head of her demons was by listening to music that made her feel good.

Anne had a different problem. Single and living alone, she checked to make sure her door was locked more times a day than she could count. Somehow, she could never believe that she had turned the knob and was safe from intruders—except when she was listening to music. The feeling of well-being that music gave her helped Anne's mind believe what her eyes told her: she had really locked the door.

Intrusive thoughts like Anne's and Lisa's can manifest in disrupted sleep patterns, poor concentration, and even lowered immunity.[21] If you have trouble feeling finished or resolved, normal signal patterns in your brain may have mutated into an unending loop.

It seems that Uplifting music can insert itself into this cycle and break the pattern. This might be because emotions can actually create thoughts, so while a low mood can generate thoughts that intrude on your sense of calm, an emotional boost can help to reinforce the message of resolution that your conscious mind is trying to send to your brain stem.[22]

Uplifting music is an easy and effective way to get the emotional kick you need to clear your mind. Research with people experiencing negative cognitions, intrusive thoughts, or dysphoria—a state of unease or mental discomfort—finds that music provides relief. After musical mood induction, people are better able to remove selected intrusive thoughts and are less threatened by stimuli that might trigger phobic reactions.[23]

Braintuning Basics: Negative or Recurrent Thoughts

....

Fill Your Mind with Music

If an uninvited thought has invaded your mind and is taking up the space you need to work, sleep, communicate, or relax, crowd it out with Uplifting music:

- Begin with focused listening to boost your mood. Follow every flip of the melody. Move to the rhythm. Sing along. Imagine the joy the musicians feel from playing together, and think back on a happy time the music makes you remember.

- When you're feeling clearer and free from negative ideas, turn the music down to play in the background, keeping you company to prevent the return of uninvited guests.

Overeating

Recent biochemical research has uncovered a connection between certain weight management problems and depression. In particular, chronic obesity seems to often be associated with shortages of serotonin, the chemical that controls the brain's satiety center and the same neurotransmitter that many depressed people lack. The popular antidepressant drug Prozac, a selective serotonin reuptake inhibitor (SSRI), increases the flow of serotonin in your brain, and doctors have discovered that treating obese people with Prozac and other serotonin stimulators like Redux can stop their food obsessions and help them lose weight.[24]

We don't have evidence that music generates serotonin (yet), but it is proven to improve your mood with physiological and brain wave arousal. So music might, like other mood boosters, help you realign your hunger with your physical needs. If you're subject to mood-related overeating, see if these braintuning techniques help.

Braintuning Basics: Overeating

Audio Appetizer

If you feel good before you sit down to eat, you won't need to rely on food for a mood boost. Try starting your meals with an audio appetizer:

- Listen to cheerful music immediately before your meal—after everything is prepared, but before you sit down. Don't begin to eat until you feel positive and energized by the music.

- If you choose to continue listening while you eat, switch to something more calming to help you slow down and enjoy your meal (see chapter 2, Relax).

Musical Dessert

It's often hard to stop eating, but it can seem impossible if your brain has failed to acknowledge that your body is full. Nearly everyone who's struggled with weight management knows that there's about a fifteen minute lag between getting full and feeling it. Try filling that gap with music.

Fifteen minutes of Uplifting selections after you've finished your meal will both boost your mood and give your brain time to catch up to your body. Think of it as dessert—a reward for taking care of yourself.

Shyness

Do you feel shy? Perhaps you have a hypersensitive amygdala, a brain circuit that controls heart rate and perspiration in reaction to stress. Or your brain might produce too much of the neurotransmitter norepinephrine, which also sends stress signals. Maybe some traumatic experiences in your past have torn at your self-confidence. Whatever the cause, if you worry that you don't know what to say or do with other people, or fear that they might be making fun of you, or get stressed out about interpersonal encounters and social occasions, you're probably shy.[25]

You're certainly not alone, though it can often feel that way. When you want to connect but are feeling self-conscious, Uplifting music can be an instant socializer.

Marilyn recalls a blind date that had her paralyzed with fear—until her roommate played Stevie Wonder's "Don't You Worry 'Bout a Thing," giving Marilyn the confidence to open the door. Jewell, a freshman in college, says the only way she can give a French presentation without getting dizzy is by listening to the disco anthem "I Will Survive" right before class.

The stimulus of musical sound has been shown to decrease shyness and increase extroversion.[26] Inducing a positive mood with Uplifting music can also enhance your performance,[27] so you can worry less. And music facilitates interpersonal relations to help make you feel like a part of the group.

Music is one of the original forms of social interaction, and an ensemble playing together in harmony is symbolic of human sharing. You've probably witnessed the magnificent social compact of an orchestra playing many parts together. You're less likely to have seen Central African hocketing in action, but it's an equally awesome exhibition of communication among people. Each participant sings or plays just one tone, so melodies are made by many people performing an interlocking succession of notes in an incredible interplay of split-second timing. It's something like a human bell choir.

Unlike language, music can be simultaneously shared by groups of people. As a listener, music can both help you prepare to be with people and enjoy yourself and them more when you're together.

Braintuning Basics: Shyness

Sound Self-Confidence

When you feel shy about a presentation or interpersonal situation, boost your self-confidence with music. Choose an Uplifting selection you love, and listen to it shortly before the nerve-racking moment. If you've made an elation tape as described earlier in this chapter and have the time to hear it through, take advantage of its benefits to feel calm but excited as you venture forth.

Social Stimulus

- **Add a soundtrack** to your social preparations by blasting Uplifting selections while you get dressed, do your hair, and so forth. Think of it as dressing up your mind.

- **Socialize your ears** with speakers, not headphones, to get accustomed to the environment of shared sound waves in the air.

• **Take your show on the road.** Listen to Uplifting music in the car on the way to your event so you arrive full of life and confidence.

The Uplift Music-Mood Checklist

❑ Uptempo, infectious beat, eighty beats per minute or more

❑ Major keys

❑ Groove

❑ Pleasing melody or hooks

❑ Harmonic consonance

❑ Simple, short, symmetrical phrases

❑ Clear, open harmonies

❑ Bright tone colors

❑ Midrange frequencies

❑ Moderate to loud volume

❑ Cooperative, jamming performance

❑ Happy, inspiring lyrics

❑ Positive personal associations

Avoid minor keys, harsh or strange sounds, downbeat tempos, introspective or solo pieces, negative lyrics, or anything you associate with feeling down.

Test Your Elation Elevation

See page 24 in the introduction for instructions on testing your music-mood response. An Uplift discography follows the quiz. Start by testing your favorite styles from the list and recording them in the journal that follows.

The Uplift Music-Mood Test

	Before Listening	After Listening	Change, Before to After
I Feel	(1–5)	(1–5)	(+ or –, 0–4)
Lively	_____	_____	_____
Interested	_____	_____	_____
Capable	_____	_____	_____
Cheerful	_____	_____	_____
Focused	_____	_____	_____
Free	_____	_____	_____
Talkative	_____	_____	_____
Playful	_____	_____	_____
Alert	_____	_____	_____
Hopeful	_____	_____	_____

Total Change:
Your Elation Elevation (0–40)   _____

The Uplift Music-Mood Journal

Date	Situation	Selection	Score

Braintuning Music: Uplift

From a world of dance music to gospel, funny songs, and feel-good rock and soul, Uplifting music swings and soars. Its catchy phrases and hooks are both familiar—for easy cognitive recognition and resulting emotional comfort—and exciting to your autonomic nervous system. The following selection includes a variety of stimulus levels, so you can find your own comfort zone.

Dance Music

Music that can get you out onto the dance floor is clearly made for feeling good—and its backbeat is like a physical lift. **Swing** into a better state of mind with **big band jazz**, **Western swing**, or **rhythm & blues**. From Count Basie to Bob Wills and the Texas Playboys, the swinging rhythmic style born in the 1920s has propelled many different dancers. Or take a detour to **ragtime, boogie woogie,** and **stride piano.** It's quieter than the big band style, but the syncopated bass lines provide a low-impact pick-me-up.

On the folksier side are the **string bands** that descend from forms like Irish jigs and reels and have accompanied American dance parties since the arrival of white settlers. Eventually spinning off into high-energy bluegrass and newgrass, string bands are a down-home way to move up the mood barometer.

The rollicking sounds of **Cajun and zydeco** from Louisiana team the waltzes and reels of the string band tradition with blues and the occasional squeeze box, or accordion. Move down to the Tex-Mex border and you'll hear similar instrumentation in **norteño** music, a mix of Mexican sounds with German polkas. Keep going south, lose the accordion, and listen to the roots of the popular song "La Bamba"—**Mexican *son jarocho*** is a shimmering mix of harp, violin, and guitars of various sizes.

From across the water in Cuba comes *conjunto*—smooth dance music with a Latin lilt. Island-hop to Jamaica and catch a positive vibe with the steady groove of **reggae**. Inspirational lyrics work with the backbeat to take your mind to higher ground.

Further afield in Africa are the infectious beat and happy cries of *soukous* from Zaire—where sweet-sounding electric guitars are used like drums in a mix of Central African music, Cuban rumba, and rock and roll. In the townships of South Africa, *mbaqanga* rocks—and accordions turn up again.

Hawaiian slack key guitar was originally based on ancient hula rhythms. Played in special tunings that contain no minor keys, the sweet sound of slack key can take you on a quick trip to sunny lands.

They've been dancing for centuries in Europe, and the **classical dance tradition** offers minuets, gavottes, sarabandes, and waltzes to stir up an elegant party in your mind.

Feel-Good Pop

Pop music has always made its mark by being upbeat, and nearly everyone has a rock, soul, hip-hop, or country song they associate with good times. Rock bands like the Beatles or the Beach Boys might never wear out their welcome. Soul began with the positive messages of the Civil Rights movement, then flowed into the handclapping tracks of Motown. Later, disco anthems took self-empowerment four-on-the-floor, and now hip-hop samples widely from all the styles of the old school. And there's a long tradition of good-time country music, from traditional groups like the Statler Brothers to the country-rock sound of Alabama.

The discography lists a few classics in each category as examples, but the possibilities are more extensive than this book can accommodate. You know what your own favorite feel-good style is. Put it on. Treat yourself.

Inspirational Music

Music made to take your spirit higher usually succeeds. Styles with the right mood traits include **gospel**, its African relative *iscathamiya*, and **choral music**. The call and response singing style of these genres creates a sense of community and togetherness—and it's good to sing along with.

Many **classical orchestra works** feature triumphal or resurrection themes that can help restore your faith. Beethoven was a master of this musical effect; several classical pieces with spine-strengthening tone are listed here.

Renaissance Music

Music of the Renaissance age, including **madrigals, chansons, and dances**, might make you think of spring and bonny lads and lasses singing tra-la. This era of renewal and optimism also saw the first printed sheet music, which brought music out of the church and royal courts and made it available for enjoyment by the masses. Perhaps that explains why in England the composers were all named "John" (Dowland, Ward, and Wilbye) and "Thomas" (Campion, Ford, Morley, and Weelkes). The light texture of Renaissance music makes it a good choice when something more insistent might make you anxious or annoyed; it's also nice for getting started in the morning and easing into your day. Choose your tracks carefully, as some music of the era has a melancholy tone.

Musicals

Show tunes tend to be upbeat and good for singing along, and also come with an associated story to take your mind off your worries. Use selected songs for quick pick-me-ups, or listen to a show all the way through when you're feeling immobilized.

Funny Songs

The cognitive power of silly lyrics can add the final touch to your musical mood boost. You won't be surprised to learn that humor can make you smile—but you might not know that it's also been shown to boost your immune system, moderate stress, and increase your sense of control,[28] which is just what you need when you're feeling low. Whether you raid the kids' record collection or prefer the quirky humor of Frank Zappa, some comical content in your music can help break a bad mood.

The Braintuning Discography: Uplift

STYLE	TITLE
Swing & Big Band Jazz	• Louis Armstrong. *Hot Fives and Sevens* Vol. 3, Columbia 44422. Though this is technically small-band and pre-swing, Satchmo's smile infuses his sound, which formed the basis for the subsequent swing era.

• Count Basie. *The Complete Decca Recordings*. Decca 3611. Big band sessions from 1937–39 by the man who defined Kansas City swing.

• *The Essential Big Bands*. Verve 17175. A compilation of the hottest bands from the swing era.

• *The Benny Goodman Quartet Featuring Charlie Christian, 1939-1941*. Columbia 45144. Goodman was one of the first to integrate his groups; getting Christian's legendary guitar on record was the happy result.

• *Fletcher Henderson 1926-1927*. Classics 705972. A pioneering arranger and bandleader of the swing era plays here with Fats Waller, Coleman Hawkins, and others. Other discs in the series span his career from 1921 to 1938.

• *"Kansas City" Soundtrack*. Verve 529554. A contemporary take on the classics featuring today's young lions.

• Glenn Miller. *Chattanooga Choo-Choo: #1 Hits*. RCA 3102. The U.S. used Miller's music in propaganda recordings during World War II. If it could turn a Nazi from Hitler to democracy, it should be enough to change your mood.

• *Django Reinhardt & Stephane Grapelli*. GNP Crescendo 9053. Gypsy guitarist Reinhardt overcame the tragedy of a fire that disfigured his hand to become a renowned virtuoso—a story as inspiring as these 1947–49 Paris sessions.

Western Swing Early Rhythm & Blues, Jump Blues	• Bob Wills & the Texas Playboys. *Anthology (1935–73)*. Rhino 70744. Wynonie Harris. *Bloodshot Eyes: The Best of Wynonie Harris*. King/Rhino 71544. • Louis Jordan. *The Best of Louis Jordan*. MCA 4079. Jumpin' tracks from 1941 to 1954 with boogie woogie rhythms and bright horn riffs. You can't frown to "Choo Choo Ch'Boogie." • Professor Longhair. *Fess: Professor Longhair Anthology*. Rhino 71502. New Orleans R&B with rolling beats and a taste of Mardi Gras.
Ragtime, Boogie Woogie & Stride Piano	• Eubie Blake. *Memories of You*. Biograph 112. This legendary pianist and composer lived to be 100; he also wrote and recorded to piano roll what might be the first song to feature a "walking" bass line. Hear it here. • James P. Johnson. *Carolina Shout*. Biograph 105. Astounding sound quality on these digital recordings of 1920s piano rolls. Fats Waller. *Fats Waller and His Buddies*. Bluebird 61005.
String Bands	• Bela Fleck. *Bela Fleck & the Flecktones*. Warner Brothers 26124. They call this banjo player the Charlie Parker of newgrass. • Jerry Douglas. *Everything Is Gonna Work Out Fine*. Rounder 11535. Bluegrass with dobro guitar. • Earl Flatt & Lester Scruggs. *Complete Mercury Sessions*. Mercury 12644. Beyond the Beverly Hillbillies. • Bill Monroe. *Country Music Hall of Fame*. MCA 10082. The grandaddy of bluegrass.
Cajun & Zydeco	• Beausoleil. *Vintage Beausoleil*. Music of the World 213. Straight-ahead Cajun dance music—a little less hectic than zydeco. • *Clifton Chenier and his Red Hot Louisiana Band in New Orleans*. GNP Crescendo 2119. Accordion-master rollicks through good-time dances. • Canray Fontenot. *Louisiana Hot Sauce, Creole Style*. Arhoolie 381.

• Queen Ida. *Cookin' With Queen Ida*, GNP Crescendo 2197. The first lady of the squeezebox.

Norteño	• *Conjunto! Texas–Mexican Border Music: Polkas de Oro*. Rounder 6051. An all-instrumental compilation featuring "polkas of gold" and spicy accordion.
Tejano	• Selena. *12 Super Éxitos*. EMI 30907. The famous Tejano-pop crossover phenomenon. Beto Villa et. al. *Tejano Roots—Formative Years*. Arhoolie 368.
Accord-ions	• *Planet Squeezebox*. Ellipsis Arts 3470. A global survey of accordion music—!
Son Jarocho	• Los Pregoneros del Puerto. *Music of Veracruz: The Sones Jarochos of Los Pregoneros del Puerto*. Rounder 5048.
Cuban Conjunto	• Orquestra Casino de la Playa. *Orquestra Casino de la Playa*. Harlequin 51 • Arsenio Rodriguez. *Los Éxitos*. Ansonia 1337. • *Mambo Fever—Ultra Lounge, Vol. 2*. Capitol 32564. The 1950s American version of Cuban dance music included maraca-shaking tracks like "Hooray for Hollywood (Cha-Cha)." Part of a 6-disc set loaded with feel-good lounge lizards.
Reggae	• Jimmy Cliff. *The Harder They Come Soundtrack*. Mango 539202. • Bob Marley & the Wailers. *Legend*. Tuff Gong 46210. Toots & the Maytals. *Funky Kingston*. Mango 539330.
Soukous Mbaqanga	• Kanda Bongo Man. *Kwassa Kwassa*. Hannibal 1343. Mahlathini & the Mahotella Queens. *Rhythm & Art*. Shanachie 43068. The original "groaner," with accordion too.
Slack Key Guitar	• Bob Brozman & Ledward Kaapana. *Kika Kila Meet Ki Ho'alu*. Dancing Cat 38031. Slack key and acoustic steel guitar duets bounce and gliss through traditional Hawaiian tunes. • George Kahumoku, Jr. *Drenched by Music*. Dancing Cat 38038. Includes vocal tracks with the wide vibrato and sweet yodels of Hawaiian singing style.
Classical Dances	• The Los Angeles Guitar Quartet. *Dances from Renaissance to Nutcracker*. Delos 3132. If the Overture to the Nutcracker Suite doesn't make you smile, try the Russian or Chinese Dance. Skip the minor mode movements. • Wolfgang Amadeus Mozart. *Serenade No. 13 in G Major ("Eine Kleine Nachtmusik") and Posthorn Serenade*. James Levine and the Vienna Philharmonic, Deutsche Grammophon 445555. Sweet

orchestral strings and the enchanting proposition of a little night music.

    • Nicolo Paganini. *Paganini for Two*. Gil Shaham and Göran Söllscher, Deutsche Grammophon 437837. Guitar and violin duets by an Italian Romantic. Try the dance and uptempo numbers (tracks 1, 3, 5, 9, 12, 14); the "Introduction and Variations" provides an iso-like build over six short movements; and the high-speed virtuosity of "Moto perpetuo" should inspire you unless you're a jealous violin player.

    • Johann Strauss. *Strauss Family Waltzes*. Arthur Fiedler & the Boston Pops. RCA Victor 61688. Triple-time classics reissued on CD.

Feel-Good Rock

    • The Allman Brothers Band. *A Decade of Hits 1969–1979*. Polydor 11156. Ten years of cruising tunes.

    • The Beatles. *1962–1966*. Capitol 97036. The years of innocence and goofy stunts.

    • Creedence Clearwater Revival. *Chronicle: 20 Greatest Hits*. Fantasy CCR-2. All the big hits, including "Proud Mary," "Down on the Corner," etc.

    • The Eagles. *Their Greatest Hits*. Asylum 105. Looking for a peaceful easy feeling?—this album recently tied with Michael Jackson's *Thriller* for the most all-time U.S. sales.

    • The Grateful Dead. *American Beauty*. Warner Brothers 1893. The band that made a nation jam.

    • Hootie & the Blowfish. *Cracked Rear View*. Atlantic 82613.

    • Little Feat. *Dixie Chicken*. Warner Brothers 2686.

Feel-Good Soul

    • *The R&B Box: 30 Years of R&B*. Rhino 71806. From Aretha to Johnny Ace, James Brown, and Jackie Wilson.

    • *Top of the Stax: 20 Greatest Hits, Vols. 1 and 2*. Stax 88005 and 88008. Everybody's here: Sam and Dave, the Staple Singers, Otis Redding, Booker T & the MGs, Johnnie Taylor—what are you waiting for?

    • Ray Charles. *Best of the Atlantic Years*. Rhino 71722. A national icon of perseverance with a smile.

    • Marvin Gaye. *15 Greatest Hits*. Tamla/Motown 6069.

    • Gloria Gaynor. *Greatest Hits*. Polydor 833433. The first disco queen sings the enduring anthem "I Will Survive."

    • The Isley Brothers. *Story, Vol. 1: Rockin' Soul*. Rhino 70908. From "Shout" to "Twist and Shout."

    • Wilson Pickett. *The Very Best of Wilson Pickett*. Rhino 71212.

    • Diana Ross & the Supremes. *Every Great #1 Hit*. Motown 5498.

    • Sam & Dave. *Best of Sam & Dave*. Atlantic 81279.

- Sly & the Family Stone. *Greatest Hits*. Epic 30325. Taking the positive message of soul into the very funky realm.
- The Temptations. *All the Million Sellers*. Motown 5212. They have sunshine on a cloudy day.

Feel-Good Country	• Alabama. *Greatest Hits*. RCA 7170. • Garth Brooks. *The Hits*. Capitol Nashville 29689. • Jimmie Dale Gilmore. *Braver Newer World*. Elektra 61836. "New country" from a man who takes himself lightly. • Waylon Jennings & Willie Nelson. *Waylon & Willie*. RCA 58401. Before there was gangsta rap, there were the original out-laws. • Lyle Lovett. *Pontiac*. MCA 42028. A tongue-in-cheek song-ster. • The Statler Brothers. *The Best of the Statler Brothers*. Mercury 822524. • Dwight Yoakam. *Just Lookin' for a Hit*. Reprise 25989.
Feel-Good Hip-Hop	• Arrested Development. *3 Years, 5 Months, and 2 Days in the Life of* . . . Chrysalis 21929. Speech adds a social conscience to the beats. • Heavy D & the Boyz. *Nuttin' But Love*. MCA/Uptown 10998. • LL Cool J. *Mama Said Knock You Out*. Def Jam 23477. • Salt 'n' Pepa. *Very Necessary*. Next Plateau/London 828392. Take a turn around the room with "Shoop."
Gospel	• *Kirk Franklin & the Family*. Gospo-Centric 72119. Contemporary arrangements and a full choir led by the exclamatory Franklin and some hard-singing soloists. • Mahalia Jackson. *Amazing Grace*. MCA 20489. The performer who defined the genre. • Sounds of Blackness. *Evolution of Gospel*. Perspective/A&M 1000. Gospel choir with a funky dance beat. • BeBe & CeCe Winans. *Heaven*. Capitol 90959. With a guest appearance by Whitney Houston. • The Winans. *Heart & Soul*. Qwest/Warner Brothers 45888. The four brothers of BeBe and CeCe are contemporary gospel favorites.
Iscatha-miya/ Mbube	• Ladysmith Black Mambazo: • *Two Worlds One Heart*. Warner Brothers 26125. The vocal group that performed on Paul Simon's *Graceland* album. • *Shaka Zulu*. Warner Brothers 25582.
Choral Music	• George Frideric Handel. The "Hallelujah Chorus" and "Amen Chorus" on *Messiah: Favorite Choruses and Arias*. Robert Shaw & the Atlanta Symphony Orchestra, Telarc 80103.

• Henry Purcell. "My Beloved Spake" and "O Sing Unto the Lord" on *Hail, Bright Cecilia!* Paul McCreesh and the Gabrieli Consort & Players, Archiv 445882. One anthem honors love, the other God, and both are rife with "alleluias."

Classical Orchestra

• Ludwig van Beethoven.

• First and fourth movement of *Symphony No. 1*. Herbert von Karajan & the Berlin Philharmonic, Deutsche Grammophon 439001. Beethoven's first symphonic work opens with a sunny feeling and a resounding finish. Want a little more?—the sprightly final movement pushes the pace.

• Fourth movement of *Symphony #9 ("Choral")*. Cristoph von Dohnányi and the Cleveland Orchestra & Chorus, Telarc 80120. This movement makes a natural iso mood vector, starting with dark, questioning phrases, weaving in themes of hope, then building into the great exultation of the famous "Ode to Joy" chorus.

• Anton Bruckner. First movement of *Symphony No. 4 ("Romantic")*. Claudio Abbado & the Vienna Philharmonic, Deutsche Grammophon 431719. Broad, big-picture music, packing sonic power without bombast.

• Gustav Holst. "Jupiter, the Bringer of Jollity" on *The Planets*. James Levine & the Chicago Symphony Orchestra, Deutsche Grammophon 429730. A bright, big, orchestral celebration of the happy planet.

• Gustav Mahler. Fourth movement of *Symphony No. 8*. Claudio Abbado & the Berlin Philharmonic, Deutsche Grammophon 445843. Like the final movement of Beethoven's Ninth, this piece for orchestra and chorus provides an iso build to a triumphal, spine-tingling finale.

• Carl Nielsen. First movement of *Symphony No. 4 ("The Inextinguishable")*. Herbert Blomstedt & the San Francisco Symphony, London 421524. Inextinguishable is how you'll feel after contrasting tone colors and harmonic surprises build into a noble assertion of firepower.

Renaissance Music

• *Ars Britannica*. Bruno Turner & the Pro Cantione Antiqua, Teldec 46004. Works by a roster of English all-stars: Byrd, Dunstable, Dowland, Ward, Wilbye, Weelkes, Morley, Campion, Ford, Pilkington, Picard.

• *The Cradle of the Renaissance: Italian Music from the Time of Da Vinci*. Hyperion 66814.

• *A Distant Mirror: Music of the 14th Century and Shakespeare's Music*. Folger Consort, Delos 1003. Delicate countertenors, recorders, and lutes float and soothe in the first half of the disc, then pick up the pace for lively works by Thomas Morley, Henry Purcell, and Thomas Arne.

• Orlando de Lassus. *Chansons & Moresche*. Ensemble Clement Janequin, Harmonia Mundi 901391. A collection of 16th-century works inspired by the *commedia dell' arte*, drinking songs, and *chansons* (French for song, though the composer was Italian), performed in a humorous manner that borders on brash. Skip the melancholy tracks: 1, 3, 5, 8, 17, 20, 21.

• *A Renaissance Tour of Europe*. New York Chamber Orchestra, Dorian 90133. Monteverdi, Hassler, Wilbye, Lassus, Morley.

• *La Rocque 'n' Roll: Popular Music of Renaissance France*. The Baltimore Consort, Dorian 90177. Rollicking numbers from Praetorius, Le Roy and the like.

Musicals
• Leonard Bernstein. *On the Town*. Michael Tilson Thomas & the London Symphony Orchestra, Deutsche Grammophon 437516. 1940s New York with a very young Bernstein.

• *"Evita"—The Complete Motion Picture Soundtrack*. Warner Brothers 46346. From the movie version.

• Gilbert & Sullivan. *The Pirates of Penzance*. Telarc 80353. Light opera.

• Rodgers & Hammerstein. *The Sound of Music—Soundtrack*. RCA 66587.

• *Singin' in the Rain*. Rhino 71963.

• Steven Sondheim. *Follies in Concert—Studio Cast*. RCA 7128.

Funny Songs
• Dr. Seuss. *The Cat in the Hat Songbook*. RCA 1095.

• P.D.Q. Bach. *1712 Overture and Other Musical Assaults*. Telarc 80210.

• The Sugarhill Gang. "Rapper's Delight" on *Best of the Sugarhill Gang*. Rhino 71986. Silly lyrics, corny handclaps, and a jamming bass line.

• Frank Zappa. *The Best of Frank Zappa: Strictly Commercial*. Rykodisc 40500.

See Page 255 for Sources.

Uplift: The Braintuning 5

A diverse sampling from the discography to get you started:

- *The Essential Big Bands*. Verve 17175.

- The Beatles. *1962–1966*. Capitol 97036.

- *Kirk Franklin & the Family*. Gospo-Centric 72119.

- Ludwig van Beethoven. *Symphony #9 ("Choral")*. Cristoph von Dohnányi and the Cleveland Orchestra & Chorus, Telarc 80120.

- Original cast. *Singin' in the Rain*. Rhino 271963.

Music Mobilizes Me

When you're feeling down, you are not alone. You're not paralyzed. You're not doomed to keep feeling this way. Music is there, within your reach, ready to get right to work on your mood and all the associated signals in your body to help you move along.

Just push Play.

Six

Cleanse

Aristotle called music medicine because it worked as a psycho-catharsis. Are you tired of trying to stay calm when you feel like you're about to explode? Try turning to music to vent your anger, frustration, and grief. You need hard music for hard times.

Cleanse Overview

Cleansing Music Can Help You With:	Use These Techniques if You Are:	How Music Helps:
Aggression	Steaming, seething—mad and ready to blow.	Provides a safe and immediate outlet for your feelings.
Repressed Anger	Snapping at people, picking fights, frustrated, or irritable.	Discharges hidden anger privately, without needless confrontations.
Grief	Recovering from a loss.	Expresses your anger, sadness, and fear to help you move on to mourning and recovery.

Problem Relationships	Preparing to or just finished talking with a boss, colleague, or relative who drives you crazy.	Gives voice to your thoughts without sharing them with their subjects, so you can stay in control.

Much has been written and said about the potential connection between hard-core music styles and aggressive or violent behaviors.[1] While these debates are important, they often overlook the fact that stormy, turbulent music is made around the world and has been for centuries. Listening to Beethoven's Fifth or the explosive *kecak* vocalizing of Bali disproves the causal connection between hard music and societies of violence, and it suggests that we make hard music to serve a vital personal and social purpose.

When anger and out-of-control emotions possess you, dramatic music can help you to ventilate your feelings and breathe easily again. Musical messages travel through the limbic system, the center of rage and fear. By helping you access these feelings at their very origin, a controlled musical catharsis can spare potential victims your wrath and save your health from the dangers of internalized fury.[2]

Anger can come from sources as diverse as a scolding from your boss to racial discrimination. It can happen when someone does you wrong or simply when you encounter a different opinion, unexpected snowstorm, or overdue bill. When you handle it right, anger can be a galvanizing force for change. But it can also be a vicious poison.

As part of the natural stress reaction that prepares you to fight and defend yourself, the emotion of anger raises your heart rate and blood pressure and releases a flow of the hormones adrenaline and noradrenaline. You're ready to do battle, even if the stimulus was nothing more than someone edging in front of you at the ATM.

High levels of anger are associated with increased risk of hypertension, heart disease, and insulin resistance syndrome.[3] There are less direct health risks, too. A recent study found a correlation between anger and smoking among women[4]—perhaps because women have fewer socially acceptable outlets for their frustrations. Anger is so powerful that it can even eat away at your sex drive, whether you're male or female.[5]

The price of unmanaged anger is high, and many psychological experts recommend constructive, private catharsis of anger to prevent lashing out at people, internalizing your feelings into your body, or letting intermittent angry explosions become part of your behavior pattern.[6]

There are other negative emotions that beg for expression, too. Grief, frustration, and fear can all be as harmful as anger if allowed to fester inside. You can't always avoid these feelings, but you can take control of your own response. Cleansing music can help you manage anger's impact on your mind, body, and behavior.

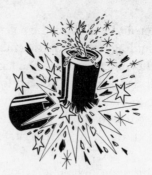

Aggression

Psychologists roughly group people into anger-in or anger-out types. Anger-out people express their feelings with assertiveness or aggression. Assertive responses to anger are considered the healthiest, allowing you both to express your feelings and resolve the situation. Aggressive behaviors, however, can hurt your personal and professional relationships, escalate your own anger response, and potentially lead to violence.

Aggression can also silently raise your cholesterol. One study found that aggressive, anger-out behavior was actually a better predictor of high cholesterol levels than other health behaviors or characteristics.[7] If anger is part of your behavior pattern, your social, professional, and physical well-being require that you find the right place to put it.

Sam is a musician who drives a limousine to pay the bills. He's the lead singer in his band and accustomed to adoring crowds and praise in his role as a performer. But not so behind the wheel of a limo. Almost without exception, Sam's limousine customers condescend to him, treating him like a servant. It's an infuriating comedown from his other life, and most of the time he drives white-knuckled with anger.

The only way Sam can get through these humiliating evenings is by filling his waiting periods with Cleansing music. He takes special driving tapes of flamenco and blues, cranks up the limo's state-of-the-art sound system, and sings along. By the time his customers return, he's forgotten their last slighting remark and can focus on the challenge of guiding a stretch vehicle through crowded night streets.

The Debate on Music and Violence

Some research and court cases link the sounds of hard music like heavy metal rock and hard-core rap to aggression, violence, drug abuse, and suicide. Findings suggesting that exposure to violent media images correlates with behavior and attitude problems, particularly among adolescent males, include these:

- A study of 2,760 fourteen- to sixteen-year-old urban adolescents found that those who listened to the radio and watched TV movies and music videos the most demonstrated more risky behaviors—drinking alcohol, smoking cigarettes and pot, cheating, stealing, cutting class, driving without permission, and having sex—regardless of race, gender, or parents' education. White males involved in five or more of these behaviors were most likely to name a heavy metal group as their favorite rock band.[8]

- Among eighty-seven adolescents, those who preferred heavy metal and rap had higher incidence of below-average school grades and behavior problems.[9]

- A study of college men watching rock music videos found that videos with violent (but nonerotic) content led to higher scores on a scale of adversarial sexual beliefs than nonviolent or erotic videos.[10] Another found that college-age males found a video rape scene to be more pornographic and sexually violent when paired with its intended soundtrack of background rock music and dialogue than when accompanied by relaxing music or viewed in silence.[11]

- A survey of African American college women found that while they considered sexually explicit rap lyrics harmful to society, they also thought they accurately represented some aspects of gender relations.[12]

However none of these investigations have found music-violence *causality*—that is, that listening to turbulent music actually leads to aggressive or self-destructive behavior. It seems more likely that angry, at-risk people have a preference for negative music, which they use not as healthy catharsis but as affirmation of their troubled state.

Furthermore, many of the controlled studies that link music to undesirable affect or behavior supplement the music with visual images.[13] These results, then, don't describe *music's* effect on people, but rather testify to the way music has been appended to television, movie, and video images to heighten the emotional experience of visual events.

The frequent incidence of rebellious or negative lyrics in hard-edged music confuses the argument. These words certainly carry a strong cognitive message, but they aren't necessarily requisite to the cathartic effect of the *music* itself. Much contemporary rap, for instance, employs antiviolence or empowering lyrics but features the same hard beats and forceful musical style as music with negative lyrical messages.[14] In both cases, the music seems to serve a cathartic purpose, suggesting that the Cleansing characteristics of musical sound are separable from the effects of its lyrics.

One factor in how Cleansing music affects you is the role that it plays in your life. If, like anger, you let it in when the situation warrants it and then move on, you're probably expressing and processing feelings in a healthy way. But just as anger is destructive as an ongoing mode, you might need to keep control of hard music's presence—and even more important, move out of it to more positive mood states.

Braintuning Basics: Aggression

Feel the Purge

To let out aggression with music, try this visualizing sequence:

- Put some Cleansing music on the stereo or Walkman and turn it up to a satisfying but safe volume. (See page 31 for information about protecting your hearing.)

- As you listen, picture the limbic system at the base of your brain, right where your spinal column connects to your head. Feel your anger originating there and flowing to all your tension spots: the back of your throat, the front of your head, your pounding heart, and knotted stomach.

- Feel the energy of the music electrify the spot where your anger begins. Imagine it as a whirling, cleansing ball of fire while it flows through and vibrates your entire limbic system. Your anger is the fuel and the music is the flame; and as the fire burns, it sucks the aggressive feelings from the far reaches of your body.

- Let the fire burn bright and hot for a moment, consuming the anger, until, with the last chord of your song, it burns itself out.

Keep It Short

When you're listening to violent music for the purpose of discharging aggression, keep it short. Extended listening can stress your body with the symptoms of hyperarousal—and might reignite your anger all over again. Stop as soon as you've dispelled your explosive sensations, and then move on to recovery.

Come Down

An important step in catharsis of any kind is returning to normal. Just as you jump in a lake or take a shower after a sauna, you should cleanse yourself of the negative feelings you express listening to Cleansing music. To come down from a Cleansing session, first listen to some calming music from chapter 2, Relax, until your heart rate has returned to normal and your emotions have subsided. You might like to follow this with a selection from chapter 5, Uplift, to return to a positive mood.

Don't skip this step! Retransitioning to calmer thoughts and behaviors helps prevent further explosions in your overexcited system.

All or Nothing or Music

It's common for anger to trigger all-or-nothing thought patterns, which rarely lend themselves to problem solving or resolution. When you find yourself presenting yourself or others with all or nothing options—"Don't go to the game tonight or I'm leaving you!"—take the third road: a break with some Cleansing music.

Jump to the Tape Player

Another typical angry cognition is jumping to conclusions. If a mild comment from a coworker has you thinking, "Conspiracy theory! They've orchestrated my downfall!" put your conclusions on hold while you jump to the tape player instead.

Catharsis in the Car

The tensions of traffic congestion can escalate to the point that they make people brandish shotguns on some city freeways. Moving vehicles can be fights waiting to happen, so keep a Cleansing selection handy in the car. When someone cuts you off in traffic, take that finger you were about to brandish and use it to press the play button. Scream along—it beats shoot-

ing, getting shot at, or having your blood pressure shoot through the sun
roof.

Excess Energy

Remember Inspector Clouseau and his murderous boss with the facial tic?
Sometimes you don't even know you're mad until your body starts to move.
Before that fidget or tic becomes a punch, slap, or unmerited barb aimed
at another person, put on some crazy music and move to it. Dance, play
air guitar, pound the floor, conduct. Don't stop until you're breathing hard
and your muscles feel spent. Listen to some Relaxing music for a cooldown
and get back to business.

Keep It in the Foreground

In general, Cleansing music makes unconstructive background listening.
The ongoing sonic and emotional onslaught is likely to put you on edge
without achieving its purpose of putting you in touch with your feelings.
This is especially important if you generally tend to be angry or sad; don't
sabotage yourself with a daily environment that brings out your darker side.

The Quick Calmer

There may be angry times when you want to skip directly to Relaxing music
and save your catharsis for later. Often, a quick calmer can help you deal
with a temper flare, slowing your pulse and giving you a moment to reassess
the situation.

Choose this option when time is short or your feelings are fleeting, but
remember the iso principle, that changing your mood with music might be
more effective when you begin with something that sounds the way that
you feel now, and *then* redirect toward your desired condition.[15] Don't stifle
intense or ongoing anger for long. It could spring up to bite you in the back
later.

Repressed Anger

Anger-in people try to swallow their feelings. With your heart beating, blood
surging, and hormones coursing, being angry without an outlet can be very
hard on your body. Health care professionals blame repressed anger for
everything from exhaustion to depression, emotional numbness, erratic explosions, hypertension, and heart attacks. Unexpressed anger can increase
your risk of physical and mental health problems and lead to resentful or
passive-aggressive behavior.[16]

Sarah is an even-tempered writer and artist who rarely raises her voice, yet she says that emotional catharsis is one of music's principal roles in her life. The Beatles and Frank Sinatra are fine for happy times, but it's Nirvana, Hole, and Soundgarden who help her purge. "I use music to explore and expunge anger, stress, anxiety, sadness, depression, grief, and general angst. Music hits me right in the solar plexus, breaks down resistance, mixes stuff up, and releases negative feelings and energy. It can clean out the gunk of modern living and leave me grounded and focused."

Mary, a mom, also likes to vent with music, but her tastes are less hardcore. "I put Phil Collins's 'I Don't Care Anymore' on endless repeat and sing along, focusing all the energy of my anger there. I keep listening until it's gone."

Many people feel compelled by societal pressures to keep their anger inside. Doing so might keep things smooth on the outside, but you'd have to be a saint to magically evaporate your negative feelings into the atmosphere. Chances are you're storing it up, and it might burst out when you snap at a coworker, sulk with your mate, get impatient with your children, or have an unexpected outburst of rage at an insignificant provocation.

If you find yourself frequently feeling resentful or irritable, there's a good chance you're suppressing anger. Let it out with music and defuse this silent killer.

Braintuning Basics: Silent Anger

Free Yourself

Angry emotions are often accompanied by a feeling of being trapped, which in turn can feed your anger even more. When your natural reactions are causing claustrophobia, music can provide a quick escape route.

Liberate yourself from anger's prison with headphones and some Cleansing music. Taking control of your environment is the first empowering step; freeing your feelings is the second. If you can, take a short brisk walk while you listen. Either way, you should return feeling refreshed, reasonable, and free.

The Hearing Habit

Do you have an unhealthy habit you use to swallow anger? Perhaps you hit the vending machine, have a drink, or light a cigarette like the women in the study mentioned earlier. Coping mechanisms are important, but some are healthier—and more expressive—than others.

If you're trying to quit one of these nasty habits, try Cleansing music to take an anger break. Tuning in instead of lighting up could add years to your life.

Fidget Less, Focus More

Anger keys up your body for action, and when you don't follow through with an expressive response, fidgeting and negative thoughts can erode your concentration.

Cleansing music stimulates your system to match the arousal of your mind, much as doctors prescribe stimulants to help control hyperactivity. In fact, rock music has been used to treat attention deficit disorder.[17] When you're tapping your toe and thinking "I can't believe he hit me with this deadline" instead of dealing with your work, music can help expel the feelings from your body so that you can regain focus in your mind. Take a five-minute Cleansing music break to give your fidgets their due, then come back with all systems go.

Express Your Feminine Fury

Evidence suggests that anger might take a higher toll on women than men.[18] From higher depression rates to worse health habits, women's anger-related woes hit hard—either because they feel anger more intensely or have fewer ways to express it. Many among us would acknowledge the female of the species as the queen of anger-in behavior.

Womenfriends, remember: It's a free country, and there's nothing unfeminine about screaming along to Nine Inch Nails.

Rage Regularly

Some suppressors admit they're so adept at denial that they often don't even know they're mad until they take a private moment to fling a vase against the wall. If repression is part of your routine, try a musical cleansing every day. It might keep some of those unexpected outbursts away.

Grief

Anyone who's spent a lonely Saturday night singing along with the blues knows that experiencing pain can actually provide some relief—and that this is one of music's strong suits.

Many cultures have traditions of musical lament, in which a certain kind of singing provides emotional release after a traumatic event, usually a death. In rural Russia, for instance, the practice is so widespread that you can hire a professional lamenter to sing on your behalf. Lamenting is also common in places as far-flung as Greece, Brazil, and Papua New Guinea, with a surprising continuity of vocal style. The tense, nasal, high-pitched characteristics of traditional laments are considered cathartic and are remarkably similar to the vocal style of some American hard rock and blues.[19]

Grief comes from loss. It's a natural reaction to losing a loved one in a breakup, move, or death. Bereavement for a failed work project or a rejected proposal is rarely talked about but real. And you might encounter sadness and loss where you least expect it—suddenly realizing that you'll never become a prima ballerina or that your mother isn't as wise as you thought she was.

Grief may be a subset of depression or its symptom or cause, and it can come accompanied with a considerable amount of anger.

Grief experts report that when a loved one dies, people will often experience anger at the victim for dying. Likewise, terminally ill patients tend to go through a period of anger toward their illness. Such emotions are especially disconcerting because they serve no functional purpose. You can't use your anger to assert yourself and request that the person not die or that the disease not kill you. The only way to let these feelings go is to experience and express them.

Bob, a college professor, talks of how the blues helped him through his grief when he lost his sister to skin cancer:

"In the first, most difficult year after losing her, listening to the blues really helped to uncork my emotions and soothe them, too. It was so perfect for what I was feeling, I could totally relate to it—not, of course, to the life of a black Southern sharecropper, but to the emotion of pain and suffering and loss. I mean the original Mississippi Delta blues, the most raw and basic, with lots of rattle and buzz and hum. And their voices! As deep and rich as their guitars, with cries and moans and yelps of pain.

"Maybe it helps that it's hard to decipher the words of many of these old blues masters, because the feeling being expressed is beyond words and rational thought."

Many people have difficulty expressing grief. In feel-good America, a problem that can't be fixed is difficult to talk about. A nonverbal form of expression like music can help to sidestep this problem. In a German hospital, for instance, music helped elderly people come to terms with their unfulfilled aims and the prospect of their own deaths.[20]

Cleansing music is a way to express the unspeakable. And when you've done so, there's a vast repertoire of uplifting music to pick up your spirits and bring back your joy.

Braintuning Basics: Grief

Tune In

Society often encourages us to avoid our pain, but psychologists say that facing it is the first step toward healing. Use focused listening sessions with Cleansing music to spend some time with your pain and give it voice.

Problem Relationships

Do you ever have the morning-after regret that comes when you've screamed at your boss, cut off a client, sworn at your mother, or fired the only person in the world who knows how your computer system works? You don't need to have an anger problem to find that there's a necessary but irritating person in your life, someone who's bound to rub you the wrong way no matter how hard you try, but who you're tied to by blood, work, or circumstance. If such relationships are long-term they're certainly worth some bilateral work on the issues between you, but often you need immediate, short-term relief.

Jeff hasn't gotten along with his boss since he passed him up for a promotion a year ago and gave the job to someone less qualified, but he's also working for the best firm in town and wants to put in another year before he moves on. So he prepares for every meeting with his boss by listening to hard-core rap, allowing himself to rage about his feelings of powerlessness to the booming bass and driving rhythm. When the music stops, he lets the anger go, flips on a soft jazz station for a minute to cool off, and goes to his meeting with a sense of control.

Sandra, on the other hand, is the eternal optimist. She expects every conversation with her mother to be pleasant and loving. But by the time she gets off the phone and her mother has made pointed inquiries about her job, boyfriend, and weight, Sandra is seething. She gets relief from grunge rock—then, with her mind clear, remembers that her mother asks annoying questions as a way of expressing love.

If your interactions with certain people always make you crazy, let Cleansing music be the receptacle for your feelings. The breathing space you gain can help you make good decisions about how to handle the relationship in the future, and the release can cut down on your daily stress.

Braintuning Basics: Problem Relationships

Preparation: Purge or Soothe?

It can be difficult to initiate a positive conversation when you bear accumulated anger toward your conversant. If you need to talk with someone who pushes your buttons, it's wise to prepare.

- Depending on the strength of your feelings, it might work best to vent your anger before the discussion. Try it once and see: Listen to one Cleansing selection, follow it with a few minutes of Relaxing music, and go to face your nemesis.

- If, however, you find that hard music before the discussion only gets you more wound up, try some Relaxing music instead to enhance your composure, and save your venting for afterward.

Aftermath: Let It Out

However you prepare for your discussion, be aware of your anger and stress symptoms as you speak. Do you feel a burn in your stomach, twinge in your muscles, contraction in your lungs, pounding in your head? Calmly observe the feelings and promise yourself to release them later. Return to your conversation. Then, as soon as you're done, hurry to your headphones and set your anger free.

As you establish the habit of purging your frustrations, you can keep your cool during difficult conversations by knowing that relief is just around the bend. Unlike primal scream therapy or kickboxing, you can keep Cleansing music in your desk, car, or backpack. Relief is only a flick of the switch away.

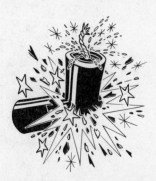

The Cleanse Music-Mood Checklist

❑ Heavy beat and rhythm

❑ Loud volume

❑ Dense or abrasive textures

❑ Noise

❑ Dissonance

❑ Minor keys

❑ Harsh or extreme tone colors—buzzing, distortion, etc.

❑ Dramatic tone

Avoid sweet, pacifying sounds or get-happy grooves. The sad selections in the discography are less turbulent than these characteristics describe; choose them for expressing sorrow or grief.

Test Your Catharsis Quotient

See page 24 in the introduction for instructions on testing your music-mood response. Notice that this test works in the opposite direction as those in other chapters. It begins by assessing your angry feelings, then measures how the music alleviates them. A Cleanse discography follows the quiz. Start by testing your favorite styles from the list and recording them in the journal that follows.

The Cleanse Music-Mood Test

	Before Listening	After Listening	Change, Before to After
I Feel	(1–5)	(1–5)	(+ or –, 0–4)
Hostile	_____	_____	_____
Clenched	_____	_____	_____
Irritable	_____	_____	_____
Abused	_____	_____	_____
Explosive	_____	_____	_____
Frustrated	_____	_____	_____
Nervous	_____	_____	_____
Overwhelmed	_____	_____	_____
Hyper	_____	_____	_____
Burning	_____	_____	_____

Total Change:
Your Catharsis Quotient (0–40)   _____
(should be negative!)

The Cleanse Music-Mood Journal

Date	Situation	Selection	Score
_____	_____	_____	_____
_____	_____	_____	_____
_____	_____	_____	_____
_____	_____	_____	_____
_____	_____	_____	_____
_____	_____	_____	_____
_____	_____	_____	_____
_____	_____	_____	_____
_____	_____	_____	_____
_____	_____	_____	_____
_____	_____	_____	_____
_____	_____	_____	_____
_____	_____	_____	_____
_____	_____	_____	_____
_____	_____	_____	_____
_____	_____	_____	_____
_____	_____	_____	_____
_____	_____	_____	_____
_____	_____	_____	_____
_____	_____	_____	_____

Braintuning Music: Cleanse

The Cleanse discography covers a wide range of musical styles to show that you don't need noise-acclimated ears to benefit from musical venting. If rock or rap is too much, try Romantic classical—or sample Spanish *flamenco*, or *rembitika*, the Greek blues. Go with whatever grabs your feelings and drags them out into the fresh air.

Hard Rock—Punk, Metal, Industrial, Alternative, Grunge

There's wide agreement, even among fans of counter-tenors and Celtic harps: Hard-driving rock is the sound when it's time to vent. Noisy guitars and rough singing seem to be the magic formula. Artist and mom Rachel names an alternative rock band as her favorite outlet for anger "because they're more pissed off than anybody." Tina, a medical researcher, vents to "anything I can scream to."

Pioneers of the distorted guitar sound include **classic rockers** like Led Zeppelin, Jimi Hendrix, and late Beatles. The roots of later hard rock styles lie here—and this can be your stopping point if the loud dissonance of later decades is too much.

Springing from the shattered dreams of the 1960s, **punk rock** was (and is) a lifestyle for some and a musical outlet for legions of people who toe the line in daily life. Jon, a brainy graduate student, favors the prototypical punk band The Fall for letting out anger. "I listen to this when I'm pissed off at authority figures, bosses, landlords, teachers, politicians, parents. This music makes me want to throw stuff, sneer, and swear at all purveyors of social bullshit."

Thrash or **speed metal** sounds like its name: fast, loud, and screaming. It took up where punk stepped back in the '80s, proving that anger isn't just a sign of the times—it's the ongoing human condition. **Grunge, industrial, and alternative rock** generally slow the beat down a touch and feature more mindful lyrics and melodic hooks.

Rap

An emphasis on lyrics that discuss issues of race, social injustice, and urban violence have made rap a natural medium for protest since it grew out of the grooves of dance DJs in the late 1970s. From the seminal days of Grandmaster Flash to the cutting edge of gangsta rap, these hard-hitting beats are perfect for dislodging those hard knots of repressed anger to let out your feelings like so many punches.

Honky-Tonk Country

The original cry-in-your-beer songs should see you through a sad jag. Better suited for private sorrow than raging anger, the original honky-tonkers had mourning down to an art.

Blues

Turn south for the front-porch approach to speaking out. The **Delta blues** are an acoustic way to work through your troubles, and, as Bob noted earlier in this chapter, are likely to be sad, buzzing, yelping—a highly personal expression of grief. Or turn up the volume and beat—and, often, turn down the pathos level—with **electric Chicago blues**. The lyrics can range from strident complaints to good-time celebrations; choose the feel that you need.

World Music

In Greece they call the blues *rembetica*. Think *bouzouki* instead of guitar, ouzo instead of whiskey, and the Mediterranean instead of the Mississippi.

Mournful modes, Gypsy sorrow, heels that stomp like a spray of bullets—*flamenco* is said to express *duende*, the soul of suffering. They called the original repertoire *cante hondo*, or deep song, for the way the music goes straight to your core and pulls out the pain with the surgical skill of virtuoso musicians.

Follow *flamenco*'s trail down to North Africa and you'll find **rai**, the incendiary Algerian and Moroccan pop style that has overcome government bans to become a worldwide sensation. Wailing vocals protest sexual and political repression while rock and roll instruments play Arabic riffs and the rhythm section gets a boost from pounding hand drums. Catharsis from people who need it.

Jewish klezmer bands echo the haunting gypsy essence of flamenco. Originally traveling musicians who roamed Russia, Poland, Romania, Hungary, and Czechoslovakia, klezmers picked up a travelogue of musical styles, and though much of their repertoire is celebratory (as can be the blues, flamenco, and so forth), klezmer's deep sense of soul and careening punk rock aesthetic (particularly in its recent revival) make it well-suited for pulling feelings out of hiding.

Cleansing music styles continue around the world. In Indonesia, heavy metal screamers have nothing on the interlocking choral style of Bali called **kecak**. This rhythmic chant, which began as accompaniment to trance dance, sounds like the yell you'd give after a swift blow to the lower abdomen. In the Korean opera tradition of **p'ansori**, every note vibrates pain through the vocal chords.

Classical

You can scream along to classical music too. Linda, a Vassar student, reports doing so to Beethoven, "and it leaves me laughing hysterically within two minutes."

Romantic opera, orchestral, and choral works are notoriously loud and emotional, and usually have the advantage of ending on a victorious note. The ninth symphonies of heavyweights Beethoven, Bruckner, and Dvorak are famously stormy, and all happened to be the composer's last. These works express the sound and fury of people preparing to meet their makers. Gustav Mahler, who as a child stated that he wanted to be a martyr when he grew up, was so fascinated by death that his music was already about fending it off just halfway through his career.

The potential downside of cleansing with a symphony is the hour or two it can take to listen. If you're in a hurry, try the first or last movement.

If you've ever spent time in church, you know that the thunder of the **organ** is bound to vibrate the demons out of your soul. Let the pipes drive your poison away.

The Braintuning Discography: Cleanse

STYLE	TITLE
Early Guitar Rock	• The Beatles. "Helter Skelter" on *The Beatles (White Album)*. Capitol 46443. • Jimi Hendrix. *Are You Experienced?* MCA 10893. • Led Zeppelin. *Led Zeppelin IV*. Atlantic 19129. • John Lennon. *Plastic Ono Band*. Capitol 46770. The first known rock album to be born out of primal scream therapy; yell along with "Well Well Well."
Pre-Punk, Punk Rock & New Wave	• The Buzzcocks. *Singles Going Steady*. IRS 13153. Fast, noisy, and with all the pop appeal of hooky tracks like "Orgasm Addict." • The Fall. *459489 A Sides*. Beggars Banquet 92380. • Iggy Pop. *Best of—Nude and Rude*. Virgin 42351. The "godfather of punk" who started it all in Detroit. • The Ramones. *Ramones Mania*. Sire 25709. Thirty tracks of non-stop drums and guitar laced with cathartic pleas like "Gimme Gimme Shock Treatment." • The Sex Pistols. *Never Mind the Bullocks, Here's the Sex Pistols*. Warner 3147. They shared their innermost feelings with the Queen of England herself.

Thrash **Metal**	• Anthrax. *Among the Living*. Island 842447. • Megadeth. *Peace Sells . . . But Who's Buying?* Capitol 46370. • Metallica. *Master of Puppets*. Elektra 60439. • Slayer. *Reign In Blood*. Def American 24131. • Soundgarden. *Superunknown*. A&M 540198.

Grunge,
Industrial,
Alterna-
tive

• Kate Bush. *Dreaming*. EMI 46361. Baroque sound complete with braying donkeys.

• P.J. Harvey. *Rid of Me*. Indigo 514696. Primal metal for thinking women.

• Hole. *Live Through This*. Geffen 24631. Courtney Love fronts this outlet for resentful grrrrls.

• Jane's Addiction. *Nothing's Shocking*. Warner Brothers 25727. With screaming guitars, tortured vocals, dissonant harmonies, and refrains like "sex is violent," the band lives up to the premise of the album's title.

• Ministry. *Psalm 69: The Way to Succeed & the Way to Suck Eggs*. Sire 26727. Heavy guitars meet dance beats—a more sociable way to rage.

• Nine Inch Nails. *Broken*. Interscope 92213. This six-song EP should contain all the thrashing noise you need; if not, check in somewhere.

• Nirvana. *Nevermind*. Geffen 24425. Buzzing guitars and throat-tearing vocals.

• Tom Waits. *Swordfishtrombones*. Island 842469. A rough, ruined voice, strange dissonance, and social angst.

Rap

• Dr. Dre. *The Chronic*. Priority 57128.

• Grandmaster Flash & the Furious Five. *Message from Beat Street: the Best of*. Rhino 71606. The first rappers to speak from the streets.

• Ice Cube. *Death Certificate*. Priority 57155.

• MC Lyte. *Bad As I Wanna B*. EastWest 61781. The first female rapper to see a single go gold. Provides one alternative to cussing out your man.

• NWA. *Straight Outta Compton*. Priority 57112. Original gangsta rap.

• Public Enemy. *Fear of a Black Planet*. Def Jam 523446. Bombastic and political.

• Queen Latifah. *Black Reign*. Motown 6370. The rapper is widely respected for her intelligent but unforgiving lyrics.

• Tupac Shakur. *All Eyez on Me*. Death Row 24204. The first double-disc rap album ever, by the late incendiary artist.

Honky-
Tonk
Country

• Patsy Cline. *12 Greatest Hits*. MCA 12.

• Merle Haggard. *Collectors Series*. Capitol 93191. Capitol sides from the 1960s and '70s such as "Tonight the Bottle Let Me Down."

• George Jones. *Hard Core Honky-Tonk—The Best of George Jones*. Mercury 848978.
• Reba McEntire. *Reba McEntire's Greatest Hits*. MCA 5979. This neo-traditionalist looks back on honky-tonk with love gone wrong songs.
• Hank Williams. *24 Greatest Hits*. Polygram 23293.

Delta Blues	• John Lee Hooker. *The Ultimate Collection (1948–90)*. Rhino 70572. He's not strictly Delta, but the eminent bluesman finds his roots there. • Son House. *Delta Blues—The Original Library of Congress Sessions from Field Recordings, 1941-42*. Biograph 118. Real down-home tracks, some recorded in a Mississippi country store, by the man who influenced Robert Johnson and Muddy Waters. • Robert Johnson. *The Complete Recordings*. Columbia 46222. The legend—and credited as an inspiration to rockers like the Rolling Stones and Eric Clapton. • Fred McDowell. *Mississippi Delta Blues*. Arhoolie 304. Bottleneck slide, 1964-65. • Charley Patton. *Founder of the Delta Blues*. Yazoo 2010. • Muddy Waters. *Complete Plantation Recordings, 1941-1942*. MCA 9344. Library of Congress field recordings made while the musician was still a sharecropper on Stovall's Plantation in the Mississippi Delta. Skip the interview tracks if they interrupt your flow.
Electric Blues	• *Chess Blues Classics, 1947–56* and *1957–67*. MCA/Chess 9369 and 9368. Celebrating the 50th anniversary of the label that recorded the first Chicago blues and went on to define the style, these collections feature Muddy Waters, Howlin' Wolf, Sonny Boy Williamson, Little Walter, John Lee Hooker, Etta James and they're digitally remastered too. • Buddy Guy. *The Very Best of Buddy Guy*, Rhino 70280. • B.B. King. *A Classic Revisited: Live at the Regal*. MCA 31106. A high-energy live set by one of America's best-loved bluesmen. • Koko Taylor. *What It Takes/The Chess Years*. MCA/Chess 9328. Few women growl like Koko, at least on record. The title track is an antidote to insults and infidelity.
Rembetica Flamenco	• *Rembetica*. Rounder 1079. • *Duende: The Passion & Dazzling Virtuosity of Flamenco*. Ellipsis Arts 3350. A 3-disc set covering traditional song, guitar virtuosos, and contemporary fusions. • *Flamenco: Fire & Grace*. Narada 63924. A compilation of today's top musicians playing in a traditional mode just this side of pop. Mostly without vocals.

• Rodrigo and Remedios Flores. *Flamenco Caravan*. Lyrichord 7424. Traditional flamenco from an Andalucían husband and wife team.
• Paco Peña. *Azahara—Flamenco Guitar Recital*. Nimbus 5116.

Rai
• Chaba Fadela & Cheb Sahraoui. *N'Sel Fik*. Blue Silver 1091.
• Cheb Kader. *The Best of Cheb Kader*. Blue Silver 1092.
• Cheb Khaled. *The Best of Cheb Khaled Vol. 1*. Blue Silver 1088. Rai's acknowledged bad boy, Khaled gets between the notes with tense, microtonal vocals.

Klezmer
• Brave Old World. *Klezmer Music*. Flying Fish 70560. Careening clarinet, killer rhythm, impassioned vocals.
• The Golden Gate Gypsy Orchestra. *The Travelling Jewish Wedding*. Rykodisc 10105.
• The Klezmatics. *Rhythm & Jews*. Flying Fish 1896–591. Raw clarinet, plaintive violin, and tracks ranging from meditative improvisations to wedding songs on speed.

Russian Laments
• *Old Believers: Songs of the Nekrasov Cossacks*. Smithsonian Folkways 40462.

Balinese Kecak
• "Sekaha Ganda Sari, Bona," on *Bali: Gamelan & Kecak*. Nonesuch 79204.

Korean P'Ansori
• *Korea: P'Ansori (Epic Vocal Art & Instrumental)*. Nonesuch 72049.

Romantic Classical
• Ludwig van Beethoven:
First movement of *Symphony No. 5*. Carlos Kleiber & the Vienna Philharmonic Orchestra, Deutsche Grammophon 447400. The well-know da-da-da-dum of the first movement can help dispel your feelings.
Symphony #9 ("Choral"). Cristoph von Dohnányi and the Cleveland Orchestra & Chorus, Telarc 80120. An emotional symphony with the famous "Ode to Joy" finale, which is your final pay-off.
First movement of *String Quartet in C minor, Op. 18, No. 4* and first movement of *String Quartet in F minor, Op. 95* on *Key to the Quartets*. The Emerson String Quartet, Deutsche Grammophon 447083. Both pieces intersperse Beethoven's darker side with melodic hope for redemption; the sound of bows sawing on gutstring is viscerally satisfying.
• Anton Bruckner. *Symphony No. 9 in D Minor*. Carlo Maria Giulini & the Vienna Philharmonic Orchestra, Deutsche Grammophon 427345. He called it his "farewell to life."
• Antonin Dvorak. *Symphony No. 9 "From the New World."* Rafael Kubelik & the Berlin Philharmonic, Deutsche Grammophon 447412.
• Gustav Mahler. *Symphony No. 6*. Pierre Boulez & the Vienna Philharmonic, Deutsche Grammophon 445835. A thundering protest against human mortality.

• Modest Mussorgsky. "Night on Bald Mountain" on *Pictures at an Exhibition and Night on Bald Mountain*. Jahni Mardjani & the Georgian Festival Orchestra, Infinity Digital/Sony 57233. This symphonic tone picture uses huge brass punches to depict Satan and his witches on the sabbath.

• Carl Orff. *Carmina Burana*. Andre Previn & the Vienna Philharmonic, Deutsche Grammophon 439950. This choral song cycle, ranging from spine-tingling to rambunctious, portrays medieval angst and the antics of salacious monks.

• Sergei Rachmaninoff. *Concerto for Piano and Orchestra No. 3 in D Minor, Op. 30*. Vladimir Ashkenazy, Bernard Haitink & the Concertbegouw Orchestra, London 417239. "Rach Three," the impassioned piece performed in the pivotal concert scene in the movie *Shine*.

• Franz Schubert. *WinterReise, Song Cycle for Voice and Piano*. Dietrich Fischer-Dieskau and Jorg Demus, Deutsche Grammophon 447421. One scholar proposes that this song cycle can be studied as a complete overview of the evolution of depression as experienced in clinical settings.[21]

• Dmitri Shostakovich:

First movement of *Symphony No. 4*. RCA Victor 60887. The pulsing strings could have served as the prototype for the shower scene music in Hitchcock's *Psycho*. The climax is as explosive as your feelings are likely to get.

Second movement of *Symphony No. 8*. Andre Previn & the London Symphony, Deutsche Grammophon 437819. Listen for the moments of machine guns firing, keeping in mind that the composer lived under the regime of Stalin.

• Igor Stravinsky. *Rite of Spring*. Pierre Boulez & the Cleveland Orchestra, Deutsche Grammophon 435769. When the ballet debuted in Paris in 1913, the audience was so aroused that fistfights broke out in the theater and the noise level rose to drown out the orchestra, leaving the dancers to go it alone.

• Richard Wagner. *The Compact Ring*. James Levine & the Metropolitan Opera Orchestra. Deutsche Grammophon 437825. Selections from the famous Ring Cycle by the composer who said that dissonance *and* women in horns were okay.

Organ Music

• Johann Sebastian Bach. "Tocatta and Fugue in D Minor" on *The Best of Bach*. Virgil Fox, RCA Victrola 60768. You'll recognize the ominous opening from scary movies. Recover with the sweet "Air" that follows.

• *Organ Fireworks I–VI*. Christopher Herrick, Hyperion. Works by a variety of composers played on the world's greatest organs: Westminster Abbey (66121) and Royal Albert Hall (66258) in

London, St. Eustache in Paris (66457), St. Bartholomew's Church
in New York (66605), Turku Cathedral in Finland (66676), and
Wellington Town Hall, New Zealand (66778).

 • *The Organ at the Cathedral of St. John the Divine—Bach, Du-
pre, Widor and Vierne.* Michael Murray, Telarc 80169. Performed in
the largest Gothic cathedral in the world. Try Dupré's "Final" for
five minutes of thunder.

For Sources see Page 255.

Cleanse: The Braintuning 5

A diverse sampling from the discography to get you started:

- The Sex Pistols. *Never Mind the Bullocks.* Warner 3147.

- NWA. *Straight Outta Compton.* Priority 57112. Original gangsta rap.

- Robert Johnson. *The Complete Recordings.* Columbia 46222.

- The Klezmatics. *Rhythm & Jews.* Flying Fish 1896–591.

- Sergei Rachmaninoff. *Concerto for Piano and Orchestra No. 3 in D
  Minor, Op. 30.* Vladimir Ashkenazy, Bernard Haitink & the Concertbegouw Orchestra, London 417239.

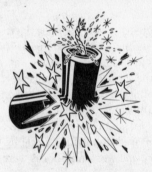

Taste the Pain

The old bluesmen sold their souls to the devil in exchange for the musical
prowess to express the pain in their souls. With Cleansing music available
on record, you don't have to. You can taste the pain and spit it out.

 Use music to exorcise your personal demons and feel the freedom of
sweet release.

Seven

....

Create

The word *music* comes from the Greek *muse*, the nine goddesses who presided over and inspired the arts and sciences. Most creativity experts agree that great ideas arise from the union of art and science . . . right and left brain . . . the rare combination of analytical and perceptual cognition that listening to music requires. When you need a muse to ignite your creative spark, what better source than music?

Create Overview

Create Music Can Help you With:	Use These Techniques To:	How Music Helps:
Problem Solving	Bring something into being, imagine, express, conceive, realize, innovate, generate, discover.	Strengthens the connection between left and right brain functions for analysis, incubation and discovery, and implementation.

Imagery	Break the limits of logic and access your right-brain intuition for inventing, artistic work, or self-expression.	Activates the right brain to spark spatial and figurative associations; provides sensory stimulation to generate images.
Productive Habits	Integrate creative thinking into your daily life for fresh approaches to work, self, and relationships.	Acts as a mood and mind cue for creative practices.

Neurologists say that we use only about 10 percent of our brains. Aren't you feeling a little shortchanged?

We may never understand or plumb the full potential of the human mind, but its ability to come up with ingenious inventions, immortal works of art, and revolutionary technologies suggests that some people push beyond that 10 percent limit. Albert Einstein and Steven Jobs must have tapped more—and maybe you can, too.

What Is Creativity?

Creativity tends to be a soft-edged term, a vague reference to the mysterious black box in which great ideas foment. For some people, creativity is the magic quality they look for in employees, colleagues, and mates; for others, the word's association with a marginalized artistic lifestyle devalues its worth.

But most creativity theorists agree that creativity is neither magical nor solely artistic. Creative thinking is instead an innate human ability that anyone can develop, and is as necessary to science, business, government, education, and sports as it is to the arts.

Inventors, businesspeople, and thinkers have developed creativity strategies for a broad array of human endeavors.[1] Their proposals for what constitutes creativity vary, but many would agree to the following components:

- Evaluation—the ability to identify problems, inconsistencies, and missing elements

- Divergent production—leaving the pack to produce something original; flexibility; fluency

- Redefinition—a sense for finding new uses for or approaches to what already exists[2]

Human creativity underlies everything from revolutionary abstract ideas to improvements in everyday procedures, and those who are able to utilize it tend to come out ahead. When you need ideas and solutions, whether it's what to serve the family for dinner or how to build a better superconductor, music can get your creative juices flowing.

Experimental evidence proves that listening to music enhances people's creativity,[3] an unsurprising discovery, but one whose potential remains largely untapped. Previous chapters of this book have described how you can use music to tap different parts of your mind, alter the state of your autonomic nervous system, and color your emotional outlook. This chapter brings together all these powers of music to demonstrate how they can help facilitate the process that sets humans apart from all other species: the creative act. It will show you how intuition and imagery—typical right-brain activities—join with analysis and logic—purview of the left brain—in the interhemispheric process of listening to music. By unleashing imagery *and* stimulating structured thinking, music can transform your natural creative power into finished works of genius like a new sales campaign, a great painting, an innovative product, or a more exciting relationship.

Problem Solving

You know the drill: old system, new needs, and you're the one who suffers from the logjam that results. The complex and changing nature of the world and the people in it requires many of us to spend a good deal of time solving problems.

Yet a surprising number of people are underprepared for this task. Many educators and creativity theorists agree that formal education in America is biased toward developing left-brain skills: language, logic, and reason. Creative, right-brain abilities like imagery, associations, analogies, and insight are often neglected in favor of sequential thinking. You need your left brain to order and analyze things, but you need an ongoing relationship between the left and right side if you ever expect to contribute anything new to the process.[4]

Your thinking habits can be as established as the way you brush your teeth. The more you memorize and restate information, the more firmly entrenched these well-worn neural pathways become. Although this might help you with your multiplication tables, the hardwired mind rarely offers the million-dollar idea.

Music, though, can redirect your neural firing to forge new pathways and add flexibility to your thought patterns. The more you branch out of your established neural networks, the more plastic your brain becomes—and the further your solutions move toward the million dollar mark.

When Hemispheres Stop Talking

Most great creative acts are the resulte of a concerted effort between both hemispheres of the brain—and communication between the sides is crucial to final output. The composer Maurice Ravel suffered from a disease that wrought progressive damage on the left hemisphere of his brain. Though his early career showed great promise and marked him as an important innovator of harmony and form, Ravel eventually lost the ability to write his music down. While he claimed to still compose in his mind—a right-brain act of imagining—he couldn't translate what he heard there into notes on paper—a symbolic, left-brain representation. Ravel's greatest works may be lost to us because his hemispheres stopped talking to each other.[5]

Listening to music can't reverse brain disease, but it can increase interhemispheric communication in healthy minds, as the processing requirements made on both sides of the brain strengthen nerve connections via the corpus callosum. Use Creating music to strengthen the pathway from your great ideas to the ability to symbolize and implement them.

Braintuning Basics: Problem Solving

The Six Questions

Six big questions[6] can help spark new ideas and focus your thoughts on any problem or challenge:

- **What** needs to be done?

- **Why** is it necessary?

- **Where** should it be done?

- **When** should it be done?

- **How** should it be done?

- **Who** should do it?

Music can provide the cue you need to ask each of these questions from a new perspective:

- Choose a song or selection for each question, and condition yourself to explore that particular query with the music.

- Use the same selections for the same questions in subsequent problems. Soon, one song will make you ask "Why?" and another "How?" without any conscious effort.

By establishing the mood for each of the big six, music can help make sure you've asked all the right questions before trying to develop the right answer.

The Four Creative Phases

Analyzing the creative process of great thinkers in many areas has led creativity specialists to break it down into four phases: preparation, incubation, illumination, and verification. The right music can help guide you through these stages for any problem or idea.

1. **Preparation—research, study, analysis:** Define the problem, need, or desire; gather information and brainstorm; set up criteria for the best solution or response. Include the big picture and ideas from other fields.

    Braintuning music: For *analysis and research*, refer to **Focus** (chapter 3), particularly the techniques for learning and recall and brainwork. *Brainstorming* is different.

    Brainstorming: This is the free-flow generation of ideas without judging them. The key is to let it rain with no umbrella; you'll get wet (have silly ideas), but you can dry off (judge and edit) later. Do this alone or in a group.

- Define and state the problem.

- Choose some music that makes you feel inspired and confident. Try improvisational styles like jazz or Middle Eastern *taqasim* (see the Create discography), and let the ongoing innovation inspire you, the occasional bad note reassure you that false steps are okay.

- Play the music and feel your mind start to rain ideas with the first sound you hear. Write down every thought without judgment, using the music as a shield against embarrassment or self-censorship.

- Let each thought trigger other ideas and associations, even if they seem tangential to the problem. If you're in a group, assign one person to write. Let other people's ideas inspire your own.

- Don't stop until the music ends. Free associate, write random words, draw pictures. Pace yourself to the musicians and push yourself to produce until they're done.

You can also use music as a right-brain primer to warm up your mind *before* you brainstorm. See the braintuning technique for abstract reasoning in chapter 3, Focus.

2. **Incubation—subconscious meditation:** Step back from the problem to process, integrate, and learn without conscious awareness. This is a downtime of not doing, surrendering, and letting go. Incubation is a Zen-like state of not thinking about your problem—tailor-made for a musical interlude.

     Braintuning music: Create (this chapter) or **Relax** (chapter 2; try the meditation techniques there).

Incubation Listening:
- Focus on the music, not your problem.

- Keep note-taking equipment on hand: paper, note cards, Post-it pads, etc. Allow yourself to write ideas if they come, but don't force it.

- Think of the music as a welcome break from the hard work of solving your problem. Congratulate yourself for completing the difficult work of preparation, and make this musical break a sign of your trust that your efforts will pay off.

- Repeat as necessary, using the same music to trigger your subconscious mind.

3. **Illumination—aha! or eureka:** Ideas suddenly arrive, whole or in part, to form the basis of your solution. Since this is an unexpected event, there's no need to schedule braintuning music. But once you've committed your revelation to paper, play your favorite tune to celebrate—the reward will motivate you to further insights in the future.

4. **Verification—implementation of the idea:** Test the results against the criteria established in phase one.

   Braintuning music: Try **Energize** (chapter 1) to generate implementation energy, and **Focus** music (chapter 3) to sharpen your wits for troubleshooting and refinement of the idea.

Long-Term Projects

If your problem-solving process extends over weeks, months, or years of time—like Einstein's theory of relativity—you might want to use a broader approach to braintuning. For a long-term puzzle, use music as a mood-dependent recall trigger:

- Pick a single CD that inspires you, and listen to it as you engage in phase one, preparation. Listen to it frequently throughout the preparation process.

- Then, encourage incubation by listening to the same recording on a regular basis: daily, weekly, or monthly, depending on the scope of your project.

- The music you heard as you gathered information about your problem will recall that knowledge at a subconscious level, rearrange it, and allow it to synthesize in new formations. Stick with your incubation listening until "Aha!" strikes.

Imitate

It's said that nothing is new under the sun, and many breakthrough ideas are modeled on old ones. This is as true in music as it is in science. During the classical age, most composers learned their craft by hand-copying the scores of the greats who came before them. Modern jazz arose when musicians took popular Tin Pan Alley songs and improvised over them. Hip-hop borrows widely from its predecessors, making the old school new.

Every field of endeavor has a continuity maintained by the practice of creative imitation, and you might find that building the better mousetrap instead of dreaming up a new creature to catch is just the solution you're after. Music can help you learn the art of imitation:

- Listen to two or more different versions of the same song or piece. Try "Bop Gun" in its original funk version by Parliament, then its hip-hop interpretation by Ice Cube. The Beatles' "I Want to Hold Your Hand" sounds very different as performed by Al Green. Compare "Mr. Tambourine Man" by the Byrds, Bob Dylan, and William Shatner. Glenn Gould's edgy piano rendition of Bach's *Well-Tempered Clavier* has an effect unlike Davitt Moroney's performance on the harpsichord. Reflect on how each artist transforms the song, applying a personal and creative mark.

- Now imagine what the song would sound like if you did your own version with a personal twist. Would you turn a classical sonata into jazz? Vintage Zeppelin into alternative rock? A Broadway tune into rap? Pick up the pace or slow it down; add or take away instruments; translate the lyrics into Japanese?

- Turn off the music and imagine what your new version would sound like. Sing or play it if you can.

- Think about what you chose to copy and what to change, and how those choices made the song yours. Now try applying these same appropriating moves to an existing product or idea.

When you listen to different versions of the same song, you force neural networks to recognize the similarities between different acoustic events (two versions of a piece in different keys might not share a single note), which primes your mind to see other relationships that don't exist on the simple physical level. This is how you move beyond mere imitation and engage in the act of creation.

Reversal

Opposites and extremes often reveal hidden nuances in objects and situations. Applying reversal to a problem can show you keys hidden by its surface. See how it works with music:

- Listen to some music and make a list of everything it's *not* (slow, rhythmic, brassy, relaxing, dissonant, plucking, soaring, etc.)

- With the same music on, repeat the exercise with your problem. Instead of widening your profit margin, how would you narrow it?

Charge lower prices, hire more staff, hold onto inventory longer? Aha! Time to invest in an inventory control system. Instead of convincing someone to sign on with the company, how would you encourage her to leave? Demote her, dock her pay, assign her to work on the least popular project . . . Hm. You haven't discussed project assignment with your candidate; maybe you can entice her to come aboard by giving her the one she likes best.

---

99 Percent Perspiration

Creativity isn't just about generating ideas; it's also about making them happen. Imagining the Sistine Chapel wasn't enough for Michelangelo. He had to paint it, too.

Realization and application are inherent to the creative process. Try Focusing and Energizing music to motivate you and organize your mind during the doing stages of your endeavors. When you come across a roadblock, take an incubation break with Create selections, or let go of frustrations with a Cleansing session. Stress is creativity's enemy, so use Relaxing or Healing music to decompress when the pressure gets high.

Imagery

The right side of the brain is the seat of direct perception—of literally seeing, rather than symbolizing or describing things. The lightbulb, which illuminates the visual field, is thus an apt symbol for the moment of "aha!" that marks many great perceptual discoveries. The visionary Albert Einstein described reaching his theory of relativity as one of those illuminating, right-brain experiences:

"During all those years there was a feeling of direction, of going straight toward something concrete [*right brain*]. It is, of course, very hard to express that feeling in words [*left brain*]; but it was decidedly the case, and clearly to be distinguished from later considerations about the rational form of the solution. Of course, behind such a direction there is always something logical [*left brain*]; but I have it in a kind of survey, in a way visually [*right brain*]."

Isaac Newton thought of gravity when he simultaneously noticed an apple falling to earth and the moon staying up in the sky. The need to integrate these disparate *visual images*—one thing falling, another not—led to his theory of gravitational force. So you could say that the discovery of gravity, which in turn sparked ideas like the laws of mechanics and mathematical analysis and modeling, was a right-brain event.

The right side of the brain is implicated in great creative work, and music can help you use it. For instance, an experiment with fifth grade boys found that background music led to higher scores on a "Thinking Creatively with Pictures" test—a measure of right-brain imagery—than did speech, industrial noise, or quiet.[7] Another study found that classical music intensified imagery and emotions for both high and low imagers.[8]

The techniques in this section are targeted to light up the right side of your mind.

Music and Your Inner Child

The great children's illustrator Maurice Sendak describes music as an indispensable element of his creative work. He praises its unique power to recall childlike fantasy; admires the way it "quickens" a drawing, and admits that music literally drags his pen across the page:

"All of my pictures are created against a background of music. More often than not, my instinctive choice of composer or musical form for the day has the galvanizing effect of making me conscious of my direction. I find something uncanny in the way a musical phrase, a sensuous vocal line, or a patch of Wagnerian color will clarify an entire approach or style for a new work. A favorite occupation of mine, some years back, was sitting in front of the record player as though possessed by a dybbuk, and allowing the music to provoke an automatic, stream-of-consciousness kind of drawing. . . . More interesting to me, and much more useful for my work, are the childhood fantasies that were reactivated by the music and explored uninhibitedly by the pen.[9]"

Sendak finds melody, harmony, and rhythm in pictures, suggesting that to the artist, the realm of the senses is one united kingdom, and music the key to its wonders.

Braintuning Basics: Imagery

Visual Listening

Combine the right-brain activities of visual thinking and music listening to empower your intuition and insight:

- Equip yourself with paper and pencil and put on some Create music.

- Draw pictures and images that describe your problem or concept: a structure, person, or object; a heart for love, firecracker for anger, etc. Use words as labels if you like, but try not to rely on them.

- Organize your drawings in a way that makes spatial sense to you. One alternative is mind-mapping, a popular creativity technique that radiates visual and spatial cues from a central idea.[10] To make a mind map of your situation, write the central idea in the middle of a large piece of paper. Then, working outward, create circles or spokes of key words, colors, symbols, icons, 3-D effects, and arrows that emanate from that idea. Let the ideas cluster as they do in your mind. Allow your map to be asymmetrical and messy, but try to be as visual as possible.

- You can also start with existing images: photographs, catalog drawings, and so forth. Start by laying them out, then draw additional pictures or associative imagery of your own.

- Another option is to storyboard your problem. Draw your situation or problem in scenes, one per note card or sheet of paper. Arrange them in rows on a wall or bulletin board so that they tell the story of what you're trying to accomplish or change. Now, start to play with the sequence. What happens if you move the first card to the end or vice versa? What if you take away or add an image? Shuffle, add, and subtract cards to spark new associations and juxtapositions.

- Use the music to stimulate and trigger your drawing. Let it guide you to draw objects from different perspectives and with different relative sizes.

- When you're done drawing or rearranging, survey your entire collection of images. Let the pictures and musical sound mix in your mind. Listen for awhile longer to see if any discoveries present themselves.

- You can further incubate your images by listening to the same music later, repeating until you've fully developed your idea or solved your problem. As both a subconscious mood trigger and an activator of right-brain thought, music can extend and deepen your perceptual process beyond the fleeting moment.

The Aha! Factor

Sometimes you can reason your way to the end of a puzzle or problem.

Other times, a moment of insight comes when you least expect it, without any introduction from your conscious mind. This is the aha! Eureka. Sudden knowing.

Sequential thinking—logic—precludes the possibility of aha! to which many inventors and thinkers attribute their greatest work. When you need to come up with something new, leave logic aside, and permit yourself the time, space, and musical support to access your intuitive power.

Sendak Drawing

If drawing or painting is your expressive medium, emulate Maurice Sendak and let music guide your pen or brush.

- Put on some Create music—maybe something that sparks your inner child or just strikes you as the mood for the day.

- Start to draw.

- Let the music move your pen. Maybe it calls up an entire scene or just a feeling or nuance. Amateur artist Jay reports that he likes to listen to John Coltrane and draw lines that follow the contours of his solo.

- Let the movement of the music quicken or bring life to your picture.

Listening on the Right Side of the Brain

Betty Edwards, author of the creativity classic *Drawing on the Right Side of the Brain*, describes how she uses the attributes of a pencil to examine a marriage.[11] She likens the pencil's gold ring to promises, the blue ring to depression in the relationship, and the yellow color to being too timid with her feelings. In the flat sides she finds a dull daily routine, but the six different facets suggest six solutions. The eraser: forgive and forget. Lead reminds her to get the lead out!—but also that if she presses too hard, it will break.

This technique, known as making attribute lists or forcing an analogy, is good for analyzing products, procedures, and, apparently, marriages. By requiring you to see relationships you might not otherwise recognize, analogies expand your perceptual range. Music processing is likewise a relational matter; here's how to use a musical attribute list to stimulate the flow of imagery:

- Listen to some music and separate the sounds in your mind. Write a list of each sound you can distinguish.

- Now, listen for the attributes or characteristics of each sound. Write them down.

- Finally, jot down any ideas the attributes spark. Be free in your associations. For instance, you might come up with something like this:

Sound	Attributes	Ideas
Drums	Hollow, thumping, beating, loud	Rhythm, repetition, pulse, groove, life
Guitar	Twanging, dry, melody, high	Pierce, penetrate, lead
Background	Full, wet, harmony, sustained	Support, filling in, richness fertility, stability

Now try this with a product, procedure, or situation in your life. See what happens.

Music As Metaphor

Similar to forced analogy, another escape from the limits of logic is metaphorical thinking—the comparison process demonstrated by phrases like *put on the back burner* or *tight as a drum*. Likening an object or idea to a dissimilar one helps you find hidden connections and take sideways leaps to break from sequential thought.

To use music to exercise your metaphorical mind, put on some music and brainstorm a list of metaphors, such as:

Saxophone like warm honey

Electric guitar like an eggbeater

Galloping rhythm

Velvety texture

Cool flutes

The chord was like standing on the edge of a cliff with rock crumbling underfoot.

- Your comparisons can be as simple or complex as you like. Don't judge them or worry about straining or extending them too far. No one will see them but you.

- Now, with the music still playing and your comparative mind primed, brainstorm some metaphors about the elements of your problem. Liken the product to a common household item, the person to a fruit, the emotion to a landscape.

In the Realm of the Senses

You can go beyond mixing sight and sound and into the full realm of the senses—the cross-sensory experience that scientists call *synesthesia*. Neurologist Oliver Sacks made the production of a physical sensation by stimulation of a different sense famous in *The Man Who Mistook His Wife for a Hat*, in which he tells the true stories of cross-sensors. Synesthetics will, for instance, see a certain color when they hear a certain sound. While such people seem to possess a unique neural wiring that literally swaps the senses, you can use your own imagination to unleash cross-sense imagery.

Creativity expert Mike Vance recommends simultaneously thinking with all five senses—what he calls *sensanation*—to broaden your creative range. You already do this when you use expressions like *a dry martini* (taste = touch), *a cold look* (sight = touch), or *a sweet melody* (sound = taste).

To listen synesthetically, try the following experiment. Put on some music. Listen for a moment and let the sound fill your ears. Now, one at a time, touch, taste, see, and smell the music.

- **Touch:** What does the music feel like? Is it soft or hard? Hot or cool? Rough or smooth or silky?

- **Taste:** Sweet, spicy, salty? Rich or clear? Crunchy? Chewy? Chocolatey?

- **Sight:** The music might be colorful or monochrome. Two- or three-dimensional. Curved, straight, jagged. Opaque or transparent.

- **Smell:** Perhaps the sound is floral. Grassy? Musky or pungent? Aromatic, like a marinara sauce at the simmer.

Listen Like Kandinsky

The Russian painter Kandinsky said he "heard" certain colors in different instruments. Here is his synesthetic palette:[12]

Flute = light blue

Cello = dark blue

Violin = green

Trumpet = red

Horn and bassoon = violet

Drums = vermilion (very bright red)

Bells = orange.

• Try listening to a classical piece using Kandinsky's color scheme. Listen for the violins first—they're easy to pick out. Close your eyes, focus on the violins' sound, and let it show you green. Maybe you see a green line that goes up and down with their melody, or a shape that expands and contracts with the music. Now add the red trumpet; perhaps it shades between the green lines, or adds red speckles or splotches or highlights, or forms a border. Listen for awhile and let the violins and trumpets paint red and green pictures for you. When you're ready, add the flutes—light blue—and keep building as long as you can juggle the instruments and colors.

• Your picture might stretch out with the music like an ongoing mural, or you can fill the page by focusing on one instrument and color at a time.

• Now open your eyes and try drawing the colors you hear with crayons, markers, or paints.

• Develop your own color palette for a favorite piece of music. For a rock song, you might see electric guitar as yellow, bass as blue, keyboard as turquoise, drums as purple, and high hat as magenta.

• Repeat this exercise, either in your mind or on paper, any time you want to access visual imagery, work with color, or stimulate sensory flow.

GIM: Gimme Peak

Inspired by the 1960s search for peak experience—the same quest for expansion of the bounds of perception that drove the psychedelic movement—music therapist Helen Bonny developed a technique called Guided Imagery in Music (GIM) to induce and explore altered states of consciousness. Bonny found that people achieved transpersonal, physical energy, aesthetic, color, symbolic, and ESP experiences—perceptual peaks—simply through music, without the psychedelic drugs popular at the time.[13]

To embark on Bonny's guided imagery journey, put on some Create music—maybe classical program music or a soundtrack—headphones, and an eyeshade. Get comfortable. And now:

- Repeat to yourself that you want to go with the music wherever it leads.

- Resist the urge to listen intellectually. Become one with the music. If you're having trouble, pick out the sound of one instrument and let it fill you up.

- Let the music carry you to its own psychic time and space.

- Allow yourself to shout, laugh, cry, or vent however the sound directs you. Let your body move without conscious commands from you.

- Watch for any symbols or feelings the music creates for you: a cave, hole, person, or path. Follow and explore them as far as you can; enter the cave, walk the path, talk to the person.

- Let the scenes of your experience change naturally. Take note of any recurrent scenes. They could represent your present problems or concerns.

- Enjoy yourself. Relax. Thrill. Peak. Then bring this expanded consciousness and your newly released store of images back to your world.[14]

Creative Productive Habits

Adopting creative habits of mind and body can make your whole life a work of invention and art. These techniques take advantage of music's unique union of logical and intuitive qualities to help you implement creative solutions in everything you do.

Braintuning Basics: Creative Productive Habits

Listen

Few insights are achieved while talking. Ancient sages and contemporary management consultants agree: You find wisdom and solutions when you stop making your own noise and open yourself to what's out there—when you listen.

When you need a break from the routine of action, stop, put on some music, and:

- Relax

- Don't do

- Attend

- Follow

- Listen

Make a Creative Space

Take a room or space in your house or office to devote to creative work. Fill it with stimulating artwork, textiles, lighting, all the tools you need—and a CD or tape player with your favorite music to create by. Have multiple copies of these recordings if you listen to them somewhere else, too; they should always be close by to take advantage of creative energy when it comes.

Portable Inspiration

You may need to engage in creative thinking outside of your designated space—in someone else's office, on a trip, etc. Take your creative mood along with a personal tape or CD player and recordings that you've come to associate with creative thinking. Listen to them whenever you need to solve a problem or make an intuitive leap.

Condition Your Creativity

In neurolinguistic programming they call it an *anchor*—an external cue that puts you into a creative frame of mind. Some creativity theorists describe it as a personal ritual. Your anchor could be a room, routine, outfit—or music.

Choose one or more musical selections to use as your creative trigger, then condition your mind to think inventively and solve problems when you hear them. Put on the music and:

- Work crossword puzzles.

- Think up ten new uses for a common household or office article you see in the room.

- Do word, math, or logic puzzles out of a book.

- Try the rec.puzzles newsgroup on the Internet.

Once you've conditioned your problem-solving mind to respond to this particular music, listen to it whenever you face a creative challenge.

I'm in the Mood to Create

In a study of music's effect on creativity, researchers found that inducing an elated or depressed mood with music resulted in significantly higher creativity measures than mood-neutral music did.[15] The lesson? The music you create by should make you feel good or bad, but not in between. Refer to Chapter 5, Uplift, and Chapter 6, Cleanse, for suggestions beyond the discography in this chapter.

"Free Your Mind, Your Ass Will Follow"

Funk songwriter George Clinton said it in a song. Boreal borrowed it as an advertisement for rock climbing shoes. The premise is solid: Let your mind loose, and the rest of your being, corporeal or otherwise, will follow close behind. Let Create music tear down any prison walls within your neural architecture.

Interrupt Yourself

An experiment that compared people's responses to unfamiliar music with their thinking habits found a correlation between mental flexibility and an appreciation for new musical styles. Independent, "low-dogmatic" subjects liked a "novel and complex audio-visual experience"—jazz music paired with a film of abstract visual images—significantly better than yielding, "high-dogmatic" subjects did.[16] While the study didn't determine direction of causality, it's a reasonable leap to propose that new music and imagery can help you maintain a flexible outlook.

Old values and belief systems limit your creativity, and new ones set it free. Things you're used to don't stimulate your mind, so you need to interrupt yourself with something new. Creativity writer Roger van Oech calls this process a "Whack on the Side of the Head",[17] while Edward de Bono dubs it "Provocative Operation".[18] It can be as easy as listening to new music.

- Start by changing the radio station. Leave what you usually listen to and dial up something new.

- Try altering your usual listening pattern. Substitute classical for rock-talk in the morning, or world music for jazz at work.

- Use the Random function on your CD player and as many discs as it will hold to keep your ears surprised.

- Make mixed tapes, sequencing selections so that each is as different as possible from the preceding one—from Yanni to Slayer, Japanese *gagaku* to chamber music.

- Stop everything in the middle of the afternoon and listen to new music for five or ten minutes.

- When you undertake a new project, open your mind by exploring a new musical style at the same time.

- Any time your thoughts seem routine, cue up something new that you've never heard before. Feel the music refresh your mind like a splash of cool water.

- When you need to make an intuitive leap, try listening to something avant garde or out there. Let the music lessen your fear of false steps—hey, this guy got a record deal!

- Start a regular CD exchange with your friends or coworkers: Pass around a few discs each month so that you always have something new on hand for your creative work. Once a disc has made the rounds, retire it and add something new to the cycle.

Stimulate Yourself

Psychological experiments have found that rats in a stimulating environment have more synaptic connections than those held in isolation, and the stimulated rodents can subsequently process more information. Another recent study with mice suggests that adequate stimulus can actually add brain cells to a fully developed adult mind. The implication is that sensory input encourages neural processing—and the more you can process, the more you can perceive.

Music is a readily available source of sensory stimulation, so listen frequently and attentively to push the bounds of your perception:

- Put on some familiar music. Perceive it as you usually do—probably as a single sum of sound.

- Now, start to listen at different levels. Try to pick out things like:

  High versus low sounds

  Melody versus harmony (background or fill)

  Individual instruments

  Fingers pulling guitar strings; the singer taking breaths, vibrating her vocal chords, and moving her mouth

  How the music builds from the bass and drums at the bottom, or the sound fills in downward, from the melody at the top

When you listen this way, you're using selective spatial attention to trigger different neural firing patterns, and now you're wired to hear this music in many different ways. As you attend to different aspects of incoming information, your perception of the stimulus becomes more sophisticated. So it is with any issue or problem. Use music to practice perceiving relationships that nobody else does, and you may find yourself owner of a new job, patent, or prize.

Monotonous Work

It would be great if life were one big creative challenge, but all too often your daily routine presents tasks that require only your physical body and some small sliver of your consciousness, leaving the rest of you irritated and bored. For tedious jobs like cleaning the house or processing paperwork, music can keep your creative, playful self engaged:

- Cue up a long piece of music with lots of emotional contrasts or a varied selection of many styles and sounds.

- Let one corner of your mind remember not to mix ammonia with bleach, or to send all new clients to the follow-up file. Turn the rest over to the music and set it free.

- If you're verbally inclined, try songs with interesting or sing-along lyrics. Simon, an English literature student, beats boredom with Bob Dylan "because his work gives me plenty to think about and analyze." Marta, on the other hand, prefers the drama of Broadway shows. "I sing along to all the parts and relive the story. Time flies."

The Three-Minute Challenge

Music, the great marker of time, can add a little pressure to your creative endeavors when you need a push. The mild stress of a musical time limit might give you just the spurt of adrenaline you need to think and act on a whole new level. To take the three-minute challenge:

- Pick a song or selection that lasts three to five minutes, and let it be your working time frame.

- Warm up by choosing a familiar object: paper clip, watering can, coffee cup. Set it in front of you. Put on your song and, while it plays, brainstorm as many new uses for the object as you can.

- Play the song again, and this time brainstorm new uses for a product, idea, service, or employee in your life.

- Use the same song for a three-minute challenge any time you need a push.

Reward Yourself

You may remember from chapter 3, Focus, that contingent presentation of music motivates people.[19] Knowing that you'll hear your favorite music after a job well done gets you going and gets results.

Use music to reward yourself for creative work. Listen to a favorite tune for:

- Each page of new ideas you generate

- Finding a fresh perspective on an old problem

- Trying something a new and better way

- Interrupting an automatic activity or thought to question it

- Thinking up a new use for something

- Each new idea implemented

Music for Mind Expansion

Travel suggests new perspectives and breaks old habits and routines, even if it's an auditory trip taken in an armchair between your stereo speakers. The different musics of the world have very distinct sounds—scales, rhythms, instruments, and forms that instantly signify the faraway lands they come from. The increased availability of world music recordings means that you can now travel the world without leaving the stereo. That's convenient when you have a meeting tomorrow and you crave a change of scene tonight.

Furthermore, unfamiliar sounds have to be freshly encoded in your brain, activating cells and creating new neural networks. While long-established circuits can handle the cadences of your favorite Stones tune, you might need to create entirely new architecture to make sense out of Japanese *Noh* music. Unfamiliar music can literally expand your mind.

- Choose something from a culture musically new to you (see the discography in this and other chapters and Sources on page 255).

- Concentrate on what you hear: What are they playing now and why? What does this have to do with what came before? What could be creating that strange clanging sound?

- Lose yourself in discovery and let your present surroundings melt away.

Living with Complexity

One of the hallmarks of a creative mind is being able to accept and live with complexity, even contradictions. Allowing complexity to exist prevents you from streamlining the best solution away.

Listening to complex or difficult music exercises your mind to allow contradictions and surprise. When simplicity starts to stifle you, try listening to some twentieth-century classical or world music to acclimate your mind to unanswered questions and mystery.

REM

Sleeping is a great way to access subconscious imagery—sometimes even in the middle of the work day.

To let go of conscious thought and give your subconscious mind free rein, follow the instructions for music-induced sleep in chapter 2, Relax. With music as an aid, you can use quick naps or semiconscious breaks to regenerate the flow of ideas at any time of day.

Oxygen, Food for the Brain

Your brain feeds on oxygen like your body does on pizza, so be sure to provide plenty when you're doing creative work:

- Precede brainstorming sessions with an Energizing selection (chapter 1), which promotes blood and oxygen flow throughout your body.

- Accompany your listening with a dance, which aids oxygenation and helps free you of inhibitions.

- Engage in regular aerobic exercise, with Energizing music to spur you along.

Love, the Food of the Senses

The ultimate act of creation is that of human life—the natural consequence of sex. Many creative geniuses have been known for their hearty sexual appetites. Don't neglect this important tool for freeing your sensory flow.

A Muse for Conjugal Creativity

Charles Darwin proposed that music was inherently sexual, a precursor of speech used by the male of the species to attract the female. This is certainly true in birds, who sing in response to a surge of testosterone. It's also true for people in many cultures. In fact, in both traditional and industrialized societies, music often serves as a socially sanctioned place to express sexuality and affirm its value to the culture and species.[20]

There's good reason for the global diffusion of love songs: Music gets inside your partner's body and sets vital processes to ticking far faster than you can hope to. The right sounds can enhance your arousal, pace your performance, and provide the variety you need to extend the delicious moment.

Some psychologists propose that people with highly developed creative powers naturally seek tension for the pleasure they get from its release,[21] which is analogous to the sexual act and also to a lot of music, especially from the Western art tradition.

The right mix of music and love is a highly subjective matter. Preferences, history, emotions, and circumstance will inevitably shape your choices. But if you aim to become a carnal maestro, here are the neurophysiological facts you need to perfect your moves with music.

- **Hit the Hypothalamus First:** In sensual matters, emotion generally precedes motion, so your first job as libidinous DJ is to access the emotional center in the limbic system to unleash the pleasure response seated there. Free your feelings with music featuring:

—Relaxed, predictable pulse to loosen tight nerves and muscles

—Warm, rich tone colors; lush textures and harmonies to stimulate the limbic system

—Steady volume and familiar sounds to make you both comfortable and focus attention on each other, not on sudden changes in the music

- **Arouse the Autonomic Apparatus:** Perhaps you prefer not to think of your erotic response as autonomic, but this is biology at work. With your respective hypothalami humming, the next step is to quicken your pulse and heighten blood pressure with:

—Quicker tempo to get your vital signs up to speed

—Louder volume to amplify the arousal effect (Break the reverie with a thrilling aria, funky groove, or brassy jazz number. You might want to dance—it scores points for romance and gets the blood flowing. When you hear a little heavy breathing, you're ready for the main event.)

• **Move to the Beat:** People began beating drums to imitate the body's natural rhythms: the heartbeat, the breath, and the procreative act. Take advantage of this ancient lesson. If you and your partner choose a mutually agreeable tempo, you can use music to synch up your bodies in an intimate tango of love.

—Find your speed zone. Not surprisingly, the heartbeat range is popular for this purpose. Witness sexy songs like R. Kelly's "Bump and Grind" (sixty-five beats per minute) or Prince's "Do Me Baby" (seventy beats per minute). Experiment—and once you've identified a few songs with the right pace for both of you, count the beats per minute and use the results as a criterion for picking additional tracks.

—Variety is the spice. Whatever your pace, mixing musical styles can extend your endurance. Just as people work out longer and harder when listening to a varied selection of music,[22] an eclectic mix could add longevity to your love.

• **Audio for the Afterglow:** Just like in a movie or book, a graceful denouement after the climax is critical to a sense of satisfaction. Even if you've just realized you're due at work in fifteen minutes, now is not the moment to crank up Soundgarden. Cool down and slow your overstimulated systems back to normal with something soft and gentle.

• **D.C. al Capo:** Like any work of art, a seductive soundtrack requires some advance planning: programming your CD player, making tapes, or perfecting your one-handed remote skills (recommended only for teetotalling paramours with a mind for disc and track numbers). When at last you hear the cry of "Maestro!" enjoy the applause, then take a tip from the top performers: D.C. al Capo (go back to the beginning and repeat as necessary).

Affirm Your Creative Power

You can draw on your verbal cognition to enhance music's creative effect by repeating one or more of the following affirmations while you listen. You might want to assign an affirmation to a specific piece of music, to spark that idea every time you hear it. Post an affirmation of the week on your CD player or Walkman. Sing the affirmation along with the song's melody, then replay it to yourself mentally at times when you can't listen to music.

- This music wakes up my natural brilliance and insight.

- I accept the unknown and the mystery of this problem, and I look forward to the surprise of its solution.

- Music is creative energy.

- I believe in new and better ways to do or view things.

- Music gives me a safe place to brainstorm and experiment with ideas.

- I believe in multiple solutions.

- I can create with as much energy and invention as the musicians I hear.

- I feel calm and relaxed about the creative act.

- Each musical idea I hear triggers an image or thought in my mind.

- Being creative gives me energy.

- Being energized makes me creative.

- Music unsticks me and sets my mind free.

- I am comfortable with every idea that crosses my mind.

- My ideas flow with the music.

- I see new perspectives and possible solutions.

- Listening to music is an adventure; I never know what will come next.

- Complexity gives me strength.

- I embrace the spirit of playfulness.

- My subconscious delivers the insight I need.

- Music helps my creativity grow.

The Create Music-Mood Checklist

❑ Surprising sounds, instruments, harmonies, rhythms, or structures

❑ Complexity

❑ Contrast

❑ Improvisation

❑ Invention

❑ Newness

❑ Happy or sad mood

❑ Dramatic, developmental forms

❑ Climactic moments

❑ Delayed resolution

❑ Varied or additive (odd-numbered) rhythms

❑ Philosophical or intriguing lyrics

Avoid predictable pop songs that throw you into familiar thinking patterns. Find what works for *you*. The creative effect of different musical styles seems to vary by gender, ethnicity, and perhaps other markers as well.[23]

Test Your Creativity Quotient

See page 24 in the introduction for instructions on testing your music-mood response. A Create discography follows the quiz. Start by testing your favorite styles from the list and recording your results in the journal that follows.

The Create Music-Mood Test

I Feel	Before Listening	After Listening	Change, Before to After
	(1–5)	(1–5)	(+ or –, 0–4)
Free	_____	_____	_____
Inspired	_____	_____	_____
Fresh	_____	_____	_____
Surprised	_____	_____	_____
Desiring	_____	_____	_____
Intuitive	_____	_____	_____
Flowing	_____	_____	_____
Curious	_____	_____	_____
Playful	_____	_____	_____
Flexible	_____	_____	_____
Questioning	_____	_____	_____
Daring	_____	_____	_____
Innovative	_____	_____	_____
Aware	_____	_____	_____
Fertile	_____	_____	_____
Open	_____	_____	_____
Seeing	_____	_____	_____
Attuned	_____	_____	_____
Colorful	_____	_____	_____
Clear	_____	_____	_____

Total Change:
Your Creativity Quotient (0–80) _____

The Create Music-Mood Journal

Date	Situation	Selection	Score
_____	_____	_____	_____
_____	_____	_____	_____
_____	_____	_____	_____
_____	_____	_____	_____
_____	_____	_____	_____
_____	_____	_____	_____
_____	_____	_____	_____
_____	_____	_____	_____
_____	_____	_____	_____
_____	_____	_____	_____
_____	_____	_____	_____
_____	_____	_____	_____
_____	_____	_____	_____
_____	_____	_____	_____
_____	_____	_____	_____
_____	_____	_____	_____
_____	_____	_____	_____
_____	_____	_____	_____
_____	_____	_____	_____
_____	_____	_____	_____
_____	_____	_____	_____

Braintuning Music: Create

All music is a product of the creative process, so anything you listen to can enrich your imagination. The discography in this chapter emphasizes music that pushes the boundaries, plays with your expectations, and surprises you into fresh ideas. Unfamiliar sounds forge new neural pathways to help you think the unthinkable. The selections are also geared toward complex music that mirrors the complications of many creative challenges and provides audible evidence of the possibility for resolution.

Also attend to the cross-references throughout the chapter for using music from other parts of the book in various creativity techniques. And remember that states of transient elation and depression can contribute to the creative process, so check out Uplift and certain Cleanse selections to move toward either end of the mood scale.

20th Century Classical

While this century might be nearly over, the sound of its art music remains new to many people. Minimalism, serialism, and an ever-broadening concept of what is harmonically consonant (versus clashing or dissonant) are some of the movements that have kept 20th-century art music new. It can be argued that Beethoven was as shocking to the people of his time as John Cage or Arnold Schoenberg have been to us—and Ludwig's present-day enshrinement in the pantheon of creative genius serves as a reminder that creativity always pushes the limits.

Classical "Program" Music

Music that tells or follows a story is good for generating imagery to expand your creative range. In classical music, such compositions can be loosely described as program music. Mussorgsky, for instance, shows you the pictures at an exhibition, Holst takes you on a tour of the solar system, and Copland depicts the rituals of spring. That should give you a new view of your subject.

Soundtracks

Music with visual associations from the big or small screen can light your right brain on fire. You can visualize the film if you've seen it before, or imagine an entirely new one. A good choice for incubation listening, soundtracks distract your conscious mind from your problem to give your subconscious room to work.

Concept & Psychedelic Rock & Funk

During the 1960s and '70s, a lot of popular music was made for the purpose of mind expansion. Drawing on science fiction, alternate modes of consciousness, and the most complex compositions yet known to popular music, artists of the psychedelic era took up where drugs left off.

Thought Rock

Add provocative, poetic lyrics to atmospheric music and you have a left–right brain challenge to get your corpus callosum in gear. Thought rock provides a good escape for your mind during incubation periods.

To Sing or Not to Sing?

Music with lyrics can stimulate your verbal imagination and trigger cognitive associations. Words and music work together to activate both sides of the brain, perhaps resulting in special interhemispheric insight. Lyrics can also enhance music's mood-inducing effect,[24] so if you're aiming for the happy or depressed states shown to support certain kinds of creativity, positive or sad words, respectively, can reinforce the mood of the music.

But verbal processing also takes place primarily in the left brain, which can (1) interfere with the analytical phase of problem-solving, and (2) distract from the right-brain imagining that can lead to intuitive leaps. So think about what you're trying to accomplish in this particular creative phase . . . Assess how attentive you are to the lyrics (you might barely notice them in very familiar or very atmospheric music) . . . And experiment with what works for you.

Composed Jazz

Duke Ellington took a creative leap when he decided to write jazz for a symphony orchestra. To wager that an improvisational, cooperative style could flourish within the orchestral hierarchy was considered a wild bet; most listeners would agree that he succeeded. Corporate executives, listen up.

Bebop Jazz

Out of 1950s beat culture sprang bebop, a jazz style that reinvented the harmonic, melodic, and rhythmic precepts of the preceding swing era. The basic idea of bebop was to improvise—make up completely new melodies on the spot—until you had explored every possibility and even touched upon the impossible. Take a turn with a Charlie Parker solo and leave the rules behind.

Free or Progressive Jazz

Like 20th century classical music, the avant garde of contemporary jazz has pushed to expand and break free of established harmonic and melodic structures. Tune in here for a great mental workout.

World Music

Any world music can surprise your mind and spur you to question your assumptions. The Create discography singles out a few styles that will take you far, far away from the Western world.

Japanese *gagaku*, or "elegant music," might be the oldest form of orchestral music on the planet. It's certainly strange to Western ears, with strident *shikurichi* oboes, droning *sho* mouth organs, pattering drums and gongs, and the surprising performance practice of heterophony. "Same difference" means that everyone plays the same tune—but differently. Individual variations in time and notes are considered part of the art. *Gagaku* is delicate, deliberate, and wildly liberating. **Noh** is Japan's classical theater music, less ritualistic than *gagaku* but equally startling.

The Middle East has a highly developed tradition of improvisation known as **taqasim**, in which virtuoso musicians compose instant melodies within the exacting framework of complex modes or *maqams*. Listen and hope that your own solution should be so inspired.

Tibetan monks, who have preserved the ancient tradition that China lost to modernization, have a unique throat chanting style that produces several notes at once. It's mesmerizing when performed *a cappella*, though Buddhists advocate the occasional honking trumpet to help nudge you toward enlightenment. Polyphonic throat singing is also found in the Central Asian mountains of Tuva.

Most cultures of the world treasure **work and fertility songs** for their productive endeavors. Let the image of procreation from the land inspire your thoughts and actions.

Contemporary **world composition** fuses native traditions with classical techniques or Western music styles to make something completely new, heard nowhere before. By experimenting with scales, instrumentation, and form and collaborating across cultural lines, these artists break rules that never even existed.

There are many more world musics easily available on record. A sampling is listed here, with more noted in other chapters of this book.

The Braintuning Discography: Create

STYLE	TITLE
20th-Century Classical	• Alban Berg. *Wozzeck*. Claudio Abbado & the Vienna Philharmonic, Deutsche Grammophon 423587. This Expressionist opera uses atonality and unusual form to tell a tragic soldier's tale.
	• John Cage. *Three Constructions*. Donald Knaack Percussion Ensemble. Rhino 70695. Famous for composing pieces of silence and writing music based on throws of the *I Ching*, Cage is considered a leader of the avant garde movement.
	• Djivan Gasparyan. *I Will Not Be Sad in This World*. Warner Brothers 25885.
	• Henryk Górecki. *Symphony No. 3* (*"Symphony of Sorrowful Songs"*). David Zinman & the London Sinfonietta, Elektra Nonesuch 79282. A haunting polyphonic setting of an old Polish prayer, a Gestapo prison song, and a folksong of mourning.
	• Erich Korngold. *Violin Concerto*. Gil Shaham, André Previn & the London Symphony Orchestra. Deutsche Grammophon 439886.
	• Olivier Messiaen. *Mystic: The Musical Visions of Olivier Messiaen*. Myung-Whun Chung & the Orchestre de l'Ópera Bastille, Deutsche Grammophon 449377. Try "Joy of the Blood of the Stars" to warm up for a brainstorm or break a creative block; it sounds like a downpour of discordant ideas, cleared by a resounding revelation at the end.
	• Steve Reich. *Different Trains/Electric Counterpoint*. Kronos Quartet & Pat Metheny, Nonesuch 79176. Real train whistles and instrumental imitations of human voices by noted string quartet and jazz guitarist.
	• Arnold Schoenberg. *Moses und Aron*. Pierre Boulez & the Royal Concertgebouw Orchestra, Deutsche Grammophon 449174. The king of serialism does opera.
	• Karlheinz Stockhausen. *Michaels Reise* (*Michael's Journey, the Soloists's Version*). ECM 21406. Michael (a trumpet) and his 9 co-players take a spare, surprising, and playful journey around the Earth.
Classical Program Music	• Aaron Copland. *Appalachian Spring*. Orpheus Chamber Orchestra, Deutsche Grammophon 427335. A ballet to celebrate the season of renewal, with themes based on a Shaker hymn.

• Hector Berlioz. *Symphonie fantastique.* Igor Markevitch & the Orchestre Lamoureux, Deutsche Grammophon 447406. One of the first programmatic symphonies ever written portrays a love affair, dreams, and witchcraft. Try it when you want to bust a genre.

• Edvard Grieg. *Peer Gynt Suites 1 & 2.* Neeme Järvi & the Gothenburg Symphony Orchestra, Deutsche Grammophon 427807. Composed to accompany Ibsen's play, Grieg's suites are packed with Scandinavian drama.

• Gustav Holst. "Uranus, the Magician" and "Neptune, the Mystic" on *The Planets.* James Levine and the Chicago Symphony Orchestra, Deutsche Grammophon 429730. The Magician conjures up the explosive side of creativity (try it to surprise yourself), while Neptune offers haunting contemplation and a few planetary bursts.

• Modest Mussorgsky. *Pictures at an Exhibition.* Jahni Mardjani & the Georgian Festival Orchestra, Infinity Digital/Sony 57233. Take a musical tour of a picture gallery that travels from the Tuileries gardens to the catacombs of Paris.

• Maurice Ravel. *Daphnis et Chloe Suite No. 2.* Paul Paray & the Detroit Symphony Orchestra, Mercury Living Presence 34306. French Impressionist ballet includes a haunting vocal chorus and broad sound imagery.

Sound-tracks

• Vijaya Anand. *Asia Classics I—Dance Raja Dance.* Luaka Bop/Warner Brothers 26847. Hindi film music from India—you have to hear it to believe it.

• Dead Can Dance. *Toward the Within.* 4 A.D. 45769. An extended song-cycle from this eclectic rock band's documentary film draws on chant, Chinese ch'in, traditional Persian song and more.

• Danny Elfman. *Edward Scissorhands: Original Motion Picture Soundtrack.* MCA 10133.

• Peter Gabriel. *Passion.* Geffen 24206. Globally inspired music for Scorsese's *Last Temptation of Christ.*

• Philip Glass. *Koyaanisqatsi Soundtrack.* Polygram 14042.

• James Horner. *Braveheart Soundtrack.* Decca/London 448295. Beloved for its bagpipes.

• Ennio Morricone. *Anthology.* Rhino 71858.

• Howard Shore. *Ed Wood: Original Soundtrack Recording.* Hollywood Records 62002. Spooky retro sounds conjure up images of monster brides and grave robbers.

• *The Sound of Light.* Narada 63914. Hans Zimmer and others contribute selections from television documentaries that travel from the dinosaurs to Columbus' voyage, Africa, and outer space.

Concept & Psychedelic Rock & Funk

• Laurie Anderson. *Big Science.* Warner Brothers 3674. The recorded version of her performance piece "United States."

• The Beatles. *Sgt. Pepper's Lonely Hearts Club Band.* Capitol 46442. Some consider it the first rock concept album.

• David Bowie. *The Rise and Fall of Ziggy Stardust and the Spiders from Mars.* Rykodisc 10134. A tale of a plastic rock star from the days when Bowie wore feather boas.

• The Byrds. *The Byrds' Greatest Hits.* Columbia 9516. Pioneers of psychedelia.

• Bootsy Collins. *Ahh . . . the Name is Bootsy, Baby!* Warner Brothers 2972. Psychedelia meets a funky groove.

• Cream. *Very Best of Cream.* A&M 3752. British psychedelic.

• Isaac Hayes. *Hot Buttered Soul.* Stax 4114. Possibly the only concept soul album ever made.

• Jefferson Airplane. *Surrealistic Pillow.* RCA 3766. Like a direct flight to San Francisco.

• Elton John. *Goodbye Yellow Brick Road.* Rocket/Island 28159.

• King Crimson. *In the Court of the Crimson King.* EG 1.

• Pink Floyd. *Dark Side of the Moon.* Capitol 46001. Tackle big issues like "time" and "money."

• The Who. *Tommy.* MCA 11417. The world's first rock opera transformed The Who from a singles pop band into concept artists.

Electronic Ambient

• Aphex Twin. *I Care Because You Do.* Sire 61790. Some consider the ambient movement a legacy of the psychedelic era. Building upon thumping drums and keyboard pads, Richard D. James gets weirder and noisier with each track.

Thought Rock

• The Costello Show (Elvis Costello). *King of America.* Rykodisc 20281. A master songwriter concentrates on his craft; liner notes penned by the artist detail the creative process behind every song.

• Bob Dylan. *Blood on the Tracks.* Columbia 33235. The artist who married thoughtful words to lyrics in the minds of many.

• Joni Mitchell. *Court and Spark.* Asylum 1001. The moody, jazz-tinged classic that brought the songwriter to fame.

• Pavement. *Crooked Rain, Crooked Rain.* Capitol 54076.

• Liz Phair. *Exile in Guyville.* Matador 51. Heavy thoughts expressed in styles from acoustic to rock and roll.

• Suzanne Vega. *Suzanne Vega.* A&M 5072. Her 1985 debut.

• The Velvet Underground. *The Best of the Velvet Underground (Words and Music of Lou Reed).* Verve 841164. Dark dream tales of street life in the '60s that laid the aesthetic groundwork for punk.

Composed Jazz

• Duke Ellington:
Black, Brown and Beige. Columbia Legacy 64274. Combines the structure of symphonic scoring with the harmonic and rhythmic innovation of jazz.

The Ellington Suites. Pablo OJC-446. An ever-astonishing procession of ideas and orchestration.

• Charles Mingus. *Mingus Mingus Mingus Mingus.* Impulse 170.

Bebop Jazz	• Dizzy Gillespie. *Complete RCA Victor Recordings 1947-1979.* RCA 66528. From his earliest recorded solos to his bebop big band, this collection includes greats like Miles Davis and Fats Navarro. • Dexter Gordon. *Our Man in Paris.* Blue Note 46394. With bebop giants Bud Powell and Kenny Clarke. • Charlie Parker. *Bird's Best Bop on Verve.* Verve 27452. '40s and '50s sessions from the famous saxman. • Bud Powell. *The Best of Bud Powell on Verve.* Verve 523392. One of the foremost pianists of his era.
Free or Progressive Jazz	• *Atlantic Jazz: The Avant Garde.* Atlantic 781709. A compilation of assumption-challenging sounds. • John Coltrane. *A Love Supreme.* Impulse! GRD-155. Coltrane called this 1964 work his gift to God; try matching the line of your drawing to his melody. • Thelonius Monk. *Monk's Music.* Original Jazz Classics 84. 1957 session with John Coltrane and Coleman Hawkins, by the man who reinvented jazz piano. • Cecil Taylor. *Unit Structures.* Capitol 84237. A leading free jazz pianist.
Asian Classical	• *Gagaku, Imperial Court Music.* Lyrichord 7126. Music from the Kyoto Imperial Court. • *Japanese Noh Music.* Lyrichord 7137. This 15th-century theater traditon offers masks and music weirder than anything in the West. • *Korea: Court Music.* Lyrichord 7206.
Middle Eastern Taqasim	• Hamza El Din. *Eclipse.* Rykodisc 10103. • Talip Özkan. *Mysteries of Turkey.* Music of the World 115. Improvisation, songs and dances performed on the Turkish *saz*, a long-necked lute. • Ali Jihad Racy & Simon Shaheen. *Taqasim:The Art of Improvisation in Arabic Music.* Lyrichord 7374. An extended improvisation on the *ud* and *buzuq*, Arab lutes.
Buddhist Chant	• *Tibetan Buddhism: Tantras of Gyuto: Mahakala & Sangwa Dupa.* Nonesuch Explorer 79198. • *Tibetan Ritual Music.* Lyrichord 7181. Chanted and played by lamas and monks in sacred temples.
Tuvan Throat Singing	• *Tuva: Voices from the Center of Asia.* Recorded, compiled, and annotated by Eduard Alekseev, Zoya Kirzig, and Ted Levin, Folkways/Smithsonian 40017.
Work, Earth & Fertility Music	• *Harvest Song: Music Around the World Inspired by Working the Land.* Ellipsis Arts 4040. Honoring the Incan rain god, the Pygmy ancestral forest, or the Georgian cult of wine; accompanying Japanese farmers in the field or the Gaelic Old Woman cutting the last

and finest sheaf, these traditional songs celebrate fertility and the productive urge.

• *Songs of the Great Lakes Indians: Honor the Earth Pow Wow.* Rykodisc 10199.

• *Voices of the Rainforest: A Day in the Life of the Kaluli People.* Rykodisc 10173.

More World Music

• Chemirani and Kiani. *Iranian Music for Zarb and Santur.* Harmonia Mundi HMA 190391. Sounds of ancient Persia.

• Baaba Maal. *Baaba Maal, Mansour Seck & Djam Leelii.* Mango 9840. West African songster sounds like the roots of the blues.

• *Trance Planet, Vols. 1–3.* Worldly/Triloka 7206, 7210, 124110. Though not really trance music as the title suggests, these global compilations sweep from Mozambique to Corsica, traditional to high tech. Never boring.

• From the palace of Yogyakarta. *The Sultan's Pleasure.* Music of the World 116. Royal Javanese gamelan for noble endeavors; try trancing out for incubation periods.

• The Necdet Yasar Ensemble. *Music of Turkey.* Music of the World 128. A 5-piece ensemble plays Sufi and Turkish classical music.

World Composition

• *Asmat Dream—New Music Indonesia Vol. I.* Lyrichord 7415. If the sound of Indonesian *gamelan* isn't adventuresome enough, try listening to it in the experimental compositions of four contemporary composers.

• *Pieces of Africa.* The Kronos Quartet, Elektra Nonesuch 79275. Renowned American string quartet collaborates with leading musicians from Zimbabwe, Morocco, Gambia, Uganda, Sudan, Ghana, and South Africa.

• Deep Forest. *Deep Forest.* Sony 57840. Sampled Baka Pygmy vocals mixed into electronic studio production.

• Nomad. *Nomad.* Australian Music International 4004. Dance music featuring the *didgeridoo* of the Australian Aboriginal musician featured on MTV Unplugged with the group Midnight Oil. Hear an original Dreaming Song set over rocking didgeridoo and drums; mix in West African drums and Native American vocals for a very nomadic experience.

Covers

• "Bop Gun." Parliament on *The Best of Parliament: Give Up the Funk,* Casablanca 526995; Ice Cube on *Lethal Injection,* Priority 53876.

• "I Want to Hold Your Hand." The Beatles on *1962–1966,* Capitol 97036; Al Green on *Cover Me Green,* Hi 107.

• "Mr. Tambourine Man." The Byrds on *The Byrds' Greatest Hits,* Columbia 9516; Bob Dylan on *Biograph,* Columbia 38830; William Shatner on *Transformed Man,* Sarabande 5614.

• Bach's *Well-Tempered Clavier* or *Goldberg Variations.* Davitt

Moroney, *Well-Tempered Clavier*, harpsichord, Harmonia Mundi 1901285; *The Goldberg Variations*, Harmonia Mundi 7901240; Glenn Gould, piano, *Gould Edition: J.S. Bach*, Sony Classical 52594.

Theta Brain-waves Sound	• Dr. Jeffrey Thompson. *Brainwave Suite: Theta*. Relaxation Company 3052. Sound pulses said to create theta waves, which are associated with creativity and imagery, accompanied by Tibetan bells, wind chimes and nature sounds.

See Page 255 for Sources.

Create: The Braintuning 5

A diverse sampling from the discography to get you started:

- Olivier Messiaen. *Mystic: The Musical Visions of Olivier Messiaen*. Myung-Whun Chung & the Orchestre de l'Ópera Bastille, Deutsche Grammophon 449377.

- The Velvet Underground. *The Best of the Velvet Underground (Words and Music of Lou Reed)*. Verve 841164.

- John Coltrane. *A Love Supreme*. Impulse/GRP 155.

- *Gagaku, Imperial Court Music*. Lyrichord 7126. Music from the Kyoto Imperial Court.

- Ali Jihad Racy & Simon Shaheen. *Taqasim: The Art of Improvisation in Arabic Music*. Lyrichord 7374.

Music Is the Answer

When you need to create something, be it a work of art or a solution, remember that before there was music there was silence.

"We poets struggle with nonbeing to force it to being.
We knock upon silence for an answering music."

—Li Po

Afterword

....

Silence

When you study music, good teachers tell you that it's the rests—the moments of silence—that define the sound.

And so it is with music in your life. Moments or hours of silence shape and strengthen the sound they surround.

Brenda, an actress, said in a *Tune Your Brain* survey, "When I'm in the car listening to too much music, I need to shut it off so I can listen to myself. It sometimes can be noise that keeps you asleep to your life."

All the braintuning applications in this book will be more effective if you treat yourself to natural pauses in your listening patterns. Fifteen minutes of quiet during the day renews music's power and prevents fatigue. An hour a week clears your auditory cortex and makes you appreciate music all the more. A day of quiet every month or year can provide an empty space for meditation and self-awareness outside of the daily bombardment of sensory stimulation.

The world is full of natural and man-made sound, from wind and birds and insects to traffic, car alarms, and electronic media. They say the only place you can experience true silence is in a hot air balloon that moves at the speed of the air around you. In this wind-driven basket, there is no discernible movement in your environment to generate sound waves.

You might substitute ear plugs or a mountain cabin for that balloon ride. Quiet, while not the same as perfect silence, is still an acceptable balance to music, speech, and noise. As you work with braintuning techniques, remember that it's silence that gives meaning to sound and maximizes music's impact on your life.

The Braintuning Glossary

Adagio: A tempo marking that translates as *at ease*, often used for the slow movements of classical symphonies, sonatas, and concertos.

Beat: The steady underlying pulse of music (most easily found by tapping your foot), usually grouped into sets of two, three, or four.

Consonance: A combination of notes whose sound wave frequencies form ratios of small whole numbers and so sound pleasing to the ears; degrees of consonance can be conditioned by culture and expectations. Consonant intervals tend to be neurophysiologically relaxing.

Dissonance: A combination of notes whose sound wave frequencies form nonintegral ratios and so sound jarring to the ear; degrees of dissonance can be conditioned by culture and expectations. Dissonant intervals tend to be neurophysiologically arousing.

Dynamics: The volume level and variations therein of a musical selection. Pop songs tend to have steady, loud dynamics, while a classical piece of the Romantic era might span a very wide dynamic range.

Form: The structure of a musical piece as determined by the patterns of its phrases, melodies, harmonies, and sections. Rock songs are often in verse-chorus-bridge form; blues tunes tend to repeat verses that follow a melodic and harmonic form of A-A-B; classical symphonies are generally structured in three or four movements, the form of each of which might vary significantly.

Harmony: The simultaneous combination of two or more notes to produce a chord. Convention, cultural conditioning, and the laws of acoustics combine to make some harmonies sound pleasing (consonant) and others harsh (dissonant), and also to create expectations for harmonic sequences in the mind.

Key: The notes (scale) and associated chords used in a piece or section of music that cause it to gravitate toward a home or tonic note—i.e., the key of C. In Western music, keys can generally be grouped into major and minor.

Melody: The sequence of tones that catches your attention and floats above the harmony and rhythm—what you would sing if you were singing along. A stepwise melody moves between adjacent tones in the scale, without big leaps up or down. Such melodies tend to sound the most smooth and natural.

Major key: Based on a scale whose notes share compatible overtones or harmonics, and so considered (by Western ears at least) the most harmonious and happy in sound. A major scale can be found on the white keys of a piano between C and C.

Meter: The pattern created by accented and unaccented beats, or how beats are grouped together. Most Western music employs meters of two, three, four, or six; odd-numbered and longer meters can be found in other music cultures. Some music, such as Gregorian chant, is unmetered, following no regular pattern of accents or grouping; other pieces, especially later classical works, might utilize varied meters.

Minor key: Based on a scale whose third tone is lowered a half-step from the major scale, creating a sad or melancholy effect to most listeners. A minor scale can be found on the white keys of a piano between A and A.

Pitch: The fundamental sound wave frequency of a tone. A bass guitar or tuba plays in a low pitch range; piccolos play high pitches.

Reverberation: The echo or lingering sound caused by sound waves bouncing off surfaces in the room. Can be electronically extended, as in a reverb box for an electric guitar.

Rhythm: The patterns made by the lengths and accents of sounds. Punk rock generally has a simple, driving rhythm, while African drumming might employ many different rhythmic patterns at once (polyrhythm). Syncopated rhythms, common in jazz, funk, rhythm and blues, hip-hop, and some rock and classical music, put the accent on weak beats, which can result in a sense of swing or groove.

Tempo: The speed music moves at and an important element of its physiological effect. Steady tempos can be measured in beats per minute.

Texture: The instrumentation of a piece and how the parts interrelate. The simplest texture is a single voice or instrument; the most complex might be a symphony orchestra. In between are rock bands and chamber groups; somewhat thicker than these are big band jazz ensembles and Balinese gamelans.

Timbre: The unique sound quality or color of an instrument or voice (think of the difference between a violin and a saxophone) determined by the series of overtones in the vibration frequencies and their patterns of onset and decay.

Sources

The Braintuning Hotline
(888) TYB-5295

Your one-stop source for all the recordings listed in *Tune Your Brain*.
Call to place credit card orders, which will be shipped directly to
you.

You can ask your record retailer to special-order recordings you don't find
in stock. You can also order recordings directly from most independent
labels by phone, fax, mail, or the Internet.

Arhoolie Records. 10341 San Pablo Ave., El Cerrito, CA 94530. (510) 525-
7471, fax (510) 525-1204.
http://www.arhoolie.com

Asylum Records. 1906 Acklen Ave., Nashville, TN 37212. Fax (615) 292-
8219.

Australian Music International. 928 Broadway, Suite 506, New York, NY 10010. (212) 253-1567, fax (212) 253-1521.
ami@ausmusic.com

Biograph Records. 35 Medford St., Suite 203, Somerville, MA 02143, (617) 627-9050, fax (617) 627-9051.
http://www.biograph.com

Capitol Records
http://www.hollywoodandvine.com

Chandos Records. Chandos House, Commerce Way, Colchester CO2 8HQ, England. +44 (0)1206-225200, fax +44 (0)1206-225201.
sales@chandos.u-net.com
http://www.chandos-records.com/

Earth Mother Productions. P.O. Box 43204, Tucson, AZ 85733. (520) 790-7061, fax (520) 886-3162.

Ellipsis Arts (also The Relaxation Company). 20 Lumber Road, Roslyn, NY 11576. (800) 788-6670, fax (516) 621-2750.
elliarts@aol.com

Fantasy Records (also Original Jazz Classics, Pablo, Prestige, and Stax). Tenth & Parker, Berkeley, CA 94710. (510) 549-2500, fax (510) 486-2015.
thinte@fantasyjazz.com
http://www.fantasyjazz.com

GNP Crescendo Records. 8400 Sunset Blvd., Los Angeles, CA 90069. (213) 656-2614, fax (213) 656-0693.
gnp@pacificnet.net
http://www.gnpcrescendo.com/

Harmonia Mundi. 2037 Granville Ave., Los Angeles, CA 90025-6103. (310) 478-1311, fax (310) 996-1389.
info@hmusa.com
http://www.harmoniamundi.com

Hyperion Records. 2037 Granville Ave., Los Angeles, CA 90025-6103. (310) 478-1311, fax (310) 996-1389.
info@hmusa.com OR info@hyperion-records.co.uk
http://www.hyperion-records.co.uk

Lyrichord Discs. 141 Perry Street, New York, NY 10015. (212) 929-8234, fax (212) 929-8245.

lyricny@interport.net
http://www.SkyWriting.com/Lyrichord

MCA Records
http://www.mca.com

Music of the World. P.O. Box 3620, Chapel Hill, NC 27515-3620. (919) 932-9600, fax (919) 932-9700.
e-mail: motw@mindspring.com
Web site: http://www.rootsworld.com/rw/motw

Narada Media. 4650 N. Port Washington Road, Milwaukee, WI 53212-1063. (800) 966-3699, (414) 961-8350, fax (414) 961-8351.
friends@narada.com

Nimbus Records
nimbuscd@aol.com

Reprise Records
http://www.Reprise.Rec.com

Rhino Records. 10635 Santa Monica Blvd., Los Angeles, CA 90025. (310) 474-4778, fax (310) 441-6575.
drrhino@rhino.com
http://www.rhino.com

Rykodisc. Shetland Park, 27 Congress St., Salem, MA 01970. (508) 744-7678, fax (508) 741-4506.
info@rykodisc.com
http://www.rykodisc.com

Smithsonian/Folkways. 414 Hungerford Drive, Suite 444, Rockville, MD 20850. (800) 410-9815, fax (301) 443-1819.
http://www.si.edu/folkways

Sparrow (also Gospo-Centric). Chordant Distribution, P.O. Box 5084, Brentwood, TN 37024. (800) 877-4443.

Telarc Records. http://www.telarc.com

Warner Brothers Records. http://www.wbr.com

Wind Records. P.O. Box 7309, Alhambra, CA 91802-7309. (800) 850-5015, fax (818) 457-6532.
pchuang@paclink.net

Notes

Introduction

[1]K. V. Hachinski and V. Hachinski, "Music and the Brain," *Canadian Medical Association Journal* 151/3 (1994): 293–5.

W. D. Keidel, "The Phenomenon of Hearing: An Interdisciplinary Discussion, II," *Naturwissenschaften* 79/8 (1992): 347–57.

[2]Jamshed J. Bharucha, "The Emergence of Auditory and Musical Cognition from Neural Nets Exposed to Environmental Constraints," paper presented at the Second International Conference on Music Perception and Cognition, UCLA, Los Angeles, CA, 1992.

Sandra Blakeslee, "The Mystery of Music: How It Works in the Brain," *New York Times* 5/16/95: B5–8.

Marilyn Chase, "Inner Music: Imagination May Play Role in How the Brain Learns Muscle Control," *Wall Street Journal* 124 (10/13/93): A1+.

Constance Holden, "Random Samples: Smart Music," *Science* 266 (1994): 968–69.

Robert Lee Hotz, "Study Finds That Mozart Makes You Smarter," *Los Angeles Times* 112 (10/14/93): A1+.

Isabelle Peretz and Jose Marais, "Music and Modularity," *Contemporary Music Review* 4 (1989): 279–93.

Peretz and Marais, "Specificity for Music," Chapter 13 in *Handbook of Neuropsychology* Vol. 8., F. Boller and J. Grafman, eds. (Elsevier Science Publishers, 1993): 373–390.

I. Peretz, R. Kolinsky, M. Tramo, R. Labrecque, C. Hublet, G. Demeurisse, and S. Belleville, "Functional Dissociations Following Bilateral Lesions of Auditory Cortex," *Brain* 117/6 (1994): 1283–301.

H. Petsche, "EEG Facilities for the Study of Brain Processes Elicited by Music and Speech," paper presented at the Second International Meeting of Pediatric Neurology, Parma, Italy, 1992.

Petsche, "EEG and Musical Thinking," paper presented at the Second Annual International Conference on Music Perception and Cognition, UCLA, Los Angeles, CA, 1992.

Frances H. Rauscher, Gordon L. Shaw, and Katherine N. Ky, "Music and Spatial Task Performance," *Nature* 365/6447 (1993): 611.

Rauscher, Shaw, and Ky, "Listening to Mozart Enhances Spatial-Temporal Reasoning: Toward a Neurophysiological Basis," *Neuroscience Letters* 185 (1995): 44–47.

Frances H. Rauscher, Gordon L. Shaw, Linda J. Levine, Katherine N. Ky, and Eric L. Wright, "Music and Spatial Task Performance: A Causal Relationship," paper presented at the American Psychological Association 102nd Annual Convention, Los Angeles, CA, 1994.

Gordon L. Shaw, Jurgen Kruger, Dennis J. Silverman, M. H. J. Aertsen Ad, Franz Aiple, and Han-Chao Liu, "Rhythmic and Patterned Neuronal Firing in Visual Cortex," *Neurological Research* 15 (1993): 46–50.

[3]Petsche, 1992a, 1992b.

[4]Blakeslee, 1995.

[5] Xiodan Leng and Gordon L. Shaw, "Toward a Neural Theory of Higher Brain Function Using Music as a Window," *Concepts in Neuroscience* 2 (1991): 229–58.

[6]Bharucha, 1992.

Robert J. Zatorre, Alan C. Evans, and Ernst Meyer, "Neural Mechanisms Underlying Melodic Perception and Memory for Pitch," *Journal of Neuroscience* 14/4 (1994): 1908–19.

[7]William H. Calvin, *How Brains Think: Evolving Intelligence, Then and Now* (New York: Basic Books, 1996).

Gerald Edelman, *Remembered Present: A Biological Theory of Consciousness* (New York: Basic Books, 1990).

[8]David Epstein, *Shaping Time* (New York: MacMillan, 1995).

[9] W. Jay Dowling, "Procedural and Declarative Knowledge in Music Cognition and Education," *Psychology and Music: The Understanding of Melody and Rhythm*, T. J. Tighe and W. J. Dowling, eds. (Hillsdale, NJ: Lawrence Erlbaum Associates, 1993): 5–18.

[10] G. Schlaug, L. Jäncke, Y. Huang, J. F. Staiger, and H. Steinmetz, "Increased Corpus Callosum Size in Musicians," *Neuropsychologia* 33/8 (1995): 1047–55.

[11]M. Polk and A. Kertesz, "Music and Language in Degenerative Disease of the Brain," *Brain and Cognition* 22/1 (1993): 98–117.

R. L. Young and T. Nettelbeck, "The Abilities of a Musical Savant and His Family," *Journal of Autism and Developmental Disorders* 25/3 (1995): 231–48.

Robert J. Zatorre, Alan C. Evans, Ernst Meyer, and Albert Gjedde, "Lateralization of Phonetic and Pitch Discrimination in Speech Processing," *Science* 256/5058 (1992): 846–9.

Zatorre, Evans, and Meyer, 1994.

[12]Rachel Nowak, "Neurobiology: Brain Center Linked to Perfect Pitch," *Science* 267 (1995): 616.

Gottfried Schlaug, Lutz Jancke, Yanxiong Huang, and Helmuth Steinmetz, "In Vivo Morphology of Interhemispheric Asymmetry and Connectivity in Eminent Musicians," paper presented at the Annual Meeting of the Society for Neuroscience, Washington, DC, 1993.

Schlaug, Jancke, Huang, and Steinmetz, "In Vivo Evidence of Structural Brain Asymmetry in Musicians," *Science* 267 (1995): 699–701.

[13]Dahlia Cohen and Roni Granot, "Cognitive Meanings of Musical Elements as Disclosed by ERP and Verbal Experiments," paper presented at the Second International Conference on Music Perception and Cognition, Los Angeles, CA, 1992.

M. S. Hough, H. J. Daniel, M. A. Snow, K. F. O'Brien, and W. G. Hume, "Gender Differences in Laterality Patterns for Speaking and Singing," *Neuropsychologia* 32/9 (1994): 1067–78.

[14]P. Anzou, F. Eustache, P. Etevenon, H. Platel, P. Rioux, J. Lambert, B. Lechevalier, E. Zarifian, and J. C. Baron, "Topographic EEG Activations During Timbre and Pitch Discrimination Tasks Using Musical Sounds," *Neuropsychologia* 33/1 (1995): 25–37.

Nicki S. Cohen, "The Use of Superimposed Rhythm to Decrease the Rate of Speech in a Brain-Damaged Adolescent," *Journal of Music Therapy* 25/2 (1988): 85–93.

C. Faienza, G. Cossu, and C. Capone, "Infant's Hemispheric Asymmetries in Perception of Music and Speech," paper presented at the Second International Meeting of Pediatric Neurology, Parma, Italy, 1992.

H. Gardner, J. Silverman, G. Denes, C. Semenza, and A. K. Rosenstiel, "Sensitivity to Musical Denotation and Connotation in Organic Patients," *Cortex* 13/3 (1977): 242–56.

Hachinski and Hachinski, 1994.

S. Hofman, C. Klein, and A. Arlazoroff, "Common Hemisphericity of Language and Music in a Musician: A Case Report," *Journal of Communication Disorders* 26/2: 73–82.

Robert Jourdain, *Music, the Brain, and Ecstasy* (New York: William Morrow, 1997).

I. Peretz, "Processing of Local and Global Musical Information by Unilaterally Brain Damaged Patients," *Brain* 113 (1990): 1185–1205.

Polk and Kertesz, 1993.

S. Samson and R. J. Zatorre, "Melodic and Harmonic Discrimination Following Unilateral Cerebral Excision," *Brain and Cognition* 7 (1988): 348–60.

Robert J. Zatorre, "Musical Perception and Cerebral Function: A Critical Review," *Music Perception* 2/2 (1984): 196–221.

R. J. Zatorre and A. R. Halpern, "Effect of Unilateral Temporal-Lobe Excision on Perception and Imagery of Songs," *Neuropsychologia* 31/3 (1993): 221–32.

[15]Hough et al., 1994.

L. L. Morton, M. J. Wojtowicz, N. H. Williams, and J. R. Kershner, "Time-of-Day-Induced Priming Effects on Verbal and Nonverbal Dichotic Tasks in Male and Female Adult Subjects," *Journal of Neuroscience* 64/1–4 (1992): 83–96.

P. San Martini, L. De Gennaro, F. Filetti, C. Lombardo, and C. Violani, "Prevalent Direction of Reflective Lateral Eye Movements and Ear Asymmetries in a Dichotic Test of Musical Chords," *Neuropsychologia* 32/12 (1994): 1515–22.

[16]Brian D. Josephson and Tethys Carpenter, "Music and Mind—A Theory of Aesthetic Dynamics," *On Self-Organization* (Springer Series in Synergetics Vol. 61, Heidelberg: Springer, 1994): 280–87.

Josephson and Carpenter, "What Can Music Tell Us About the Nature of the Mind? A Platonic Model," *Proceedings of Toward A Scientific Basis for Consciousness* (Cambridge, MA, IP).

[17]Roger Hyde, "Priests of Another Knowledge," *Whole Earth Review* (Spring 1996): 95–99.

[18]C. Furman, "The Effect of Musical Stimulation on the Brainwave Production of Children," *Journal of Music Therapy* 15 (1978): 108–17.

[19]I. M. Hyde, "Effects of Music Upon Electrocardiograms and Blood Pressure," *Journal of Experimental Psychology* 7 (1924): 213–24.

[20]G. Harrer and H. Harrer, "Music, Emotion and Autonomic Function," *Music and the Brain: Studies in the Neurology of Music,* MacDonald Critchley and R. A. Henson, eds. (London: Heinemann, 1977), 202–16.

Carol A. Smith and Larry W. Morris, "The Effects of Stimulative and Sedative Music on Cognitive and Emotional Components of Anxiety," *Psychological Reports* 38/3 (1976): 1187–93.

Smith and Morris, "Differential Effects of Stimulative and Sedative Music on Anxiety, Concentration, and Performance," *Psychological Reports* 41/3 (1977): 1047–53.

Jayne M. Standley, "Music Research in Medical/Dental Treatment: Meta-Analyses and Clinical Applications," *Journal of Music Therapy* 23/2 (1986): 56–122.

Michael Thaut, Sandra Schleiffers, and William Davis, "Analysis of the EMG Activity in Biceps and Triceps Muscle in an Upper Extremity Gross Motor Task under the Influence of Auditory Rhythm," *Journal of Music Therapy* 28/2 (1991): 64–88.

S. D. VanderArk and D. Ely, "Biochemical and Galvanic Skin Responses to Music Stimuli by College Students in Biology and Music," *Perceptual and Motor Skills* 74/3 (1992): 1079–90.

VanderArk and Ely, "Cortisol, Biochemical, and Galvanic Skin Responses to Music Stimuli of Different Preference Values by College Students in Biology and Music," *Perceptual and Motor Skills* 77/1 (1993): 227–34.

[21]Mark S. Rider, Joe W. Floyd, and Jay Kirkpatrick, "The Effect of Music, Imagery, and Relaxation on Adrenal Corticosteroids and the Re-entrainment of Circadian Rhythms," *Journal of Music Therapy* 22 (1985): 46–58.

[22]Samuel J. Mathews, *On the Effects of Music in Curing and Palliating Diseases* (Philadelphia: P. K. Wagner, 1806).

[23]J. Altschuler, "A Psychiatrist's Experiences with Music as a Therapeutic Agent," *Music and Medicine*, S. Schullian and H. Schoer, eds. (New York: Schuman, 1948): 96–102.

E. L. Gatewood, "The Psychology of Music in Relation to Anesthesia," *American Journal of Surgical Anesthesia* 35 (1921): 47–50.

George N. Heller, "Ideas, Initiatives, and Implementations: Music Therapy in America, 1789–1848," *Journal of Music Therapy* 24/1 (1987): 35–46.

Michael Pignatiello, Lee Anna Rasar, and Cameron J. Camp, "Musical Mood Induction: An Alternative to the Velten Technique," *Journal of Abnormal Psychology* 95/3 (1986): 295–97.

Michael Pignatiello, Cameron J. Camp, S. Thomas Elder, and Lee Anna

Rasar, "A Psychophysiological Comparison of the Velten and Musical Mood Induction Techniques," *Journal of Music Therapy* 26/3 (1989): 140–54.

L. Shatin, "Alteration of Mood via Music: A Study of the Vectoring Effect," *Journal of Psychology* 75/1 (1970): 81–86.

[24]Jill E. Adaman and Paul H. Blaney, "The Effects of Musical Mood Induction on Creativity," *Journal of Creative Behavior* 29/2 (1995): 95–108.

J. D. Brown and T. A. Mankowski, "Self-Esteem, Mood, and Self-Evaluation: Changes in Mood and the Way You See You," *Journal of Personality and Social Psychology* 64/3 (1993): 421–30.

Geoffrey L. Collier, "Emotional Responses to Music: A Three Component Model," paper presented at the Annual Conference of the Society for Music Perception and Cognition, Philadelphia, PA, 1993.

Shelley Katsh and Carol Merle-Fishman, *The Music Within You* (New York: Fireside, 1985).

Pignatiello, Camp, Elder, and Rasar, 1989.

B. L. Wheeler, "Relationship of Personal Characteristics to Mood and Enjoyment After Hearing Live and Recorded Music and to Musical Taste," *Psychology of Music* 13/2 (1985): 81–92.

C. Robazza, C. Macaluso, and V. D'Urso, "Emotional Reactions to Music by Gender, Age, and Expertise," *Perceptual and Motor Skills* 79/2 (1994): 939–44.

[25]Charles Burney, *A General History of Music from the Earliest Ages to the Present Period* (London: Oxford University Press, 1935, orig. 1789).

Emil Gutheil, ed., *Music and Your Emotions* (New York: Liveright Publishing Corporation, 1952).

Heller, 1987.

Standley, 1986.

Dorothy M. Schullian and Max Schoen, eds., *Music and Medicine* (New York: Henry Schuman, 1948).

Anthony Storr, *Music and the Mind* (New York: The Free Press, 1992).

[26] Heller, 1987.

Hyde, 1924.

S. Munroe and B. Mount, "Music Therapy in Palliative Care," *CMA Journal* 119 (1978): 1029–34.

Edward Podolsky, M.D., *The Doctor Prescribes Music: The Influence of Music on Health and Personality* (New York: Frederick A. Stokes Company, 1939).

Standley, 1986.

[27]M. Iwanaga, "Relationship Between Heart Rate and Preference for Tempo of Music," *Perceptual and Motor Skills* 81/2 (1995): 435–40.

Terence McLaughlin, *Music and Communication* (New York: St. Martin's Press, 1970): 31–34.

Curt Sachs, *Rhythm and Tempo* (London: Dent, 1953).

[28]W. B. Davis and M. H. Thaut, "The Influence of Preferred Relaxing Music on Measures of State Anxiety, Relaxation, and Physiological Responses," *Journal of Music Therapy* 26 (1989): 168–87.

Harrer and Harrer, 1977.

Standley, 1986.

P. Updike, "Music Therapy Results for ICU Patients," *Dimensions of Critical Care Nursing* 9 (1990): 39–45.

VanderArk and Ely, 1992, 1993.

Wheeler, 1985.

[29]Albert Leblanc, "An Interactive Theory of Music Preference," *Journal of Music Therapy* 19/1 (1982): 28–45.

[30]D. Fucci, D. Harris, L. Petrosino, and M. Banks, "The Effect of Preference for Rock Music on Magnitude-Estimation Scaling Behavior in Young Adults," *Perceptual and Motor Skills* 76/3 (1993): 1171–76.

Fucci, Harris, Petrosino, and Banks, "Effect of Preference for Rock Music on Magnitude-Production Scaling Behavior in Young Adults: A Validation," *Perceptual and Motor Skills* 77/3 (1993): 811–15.

D. Fucci, L. Petrosino, and M. Banks, "Effects of Gender and Listeners' Preference on Magnitude-Estimation Scaling of Rock Music," *Perceptual and Motor Skills* 78/3 (1994): 1235–42.

[31]P. O. Peretti and K. Swenson, "Effects of Music on Anxiety as Determined by Physiological Skin Responses," *Research in Music Education* 22 (1974): 278–83.

VanderArk and Ely, 1992, 1993.

Chapter One

[1]Pignatiello, Camp, Elder, and Rasar, 1989.

Smith and Morris, 1976, 1977.

Thaut, Schleiffers, and Davis, 1991.

VanderArk and Ely, 1992, 1993.

[2] Furman, 1978.

[3] John M. Geringer, "Tuning Preferences in Recorded Orchestral Music," *Journal of Research in Music Education* 24 (1976): 169–76.

Wendy L. Sims, "Effect of Tempo on Music Preference of Preschool through Fourth-Grade Children," *Applications of Research in Music Behavior,*

Clifford K. Madsen and Carol A. Prickett, eds. (Tuscaloosa and London: The University of Alabama Press, 1987): 15–25.

J. Wapnick, "Pitch, Tempo, and Timbral Preferences in Recorded Piano Music," *Journal of Research in Music Education* 28 (1980): 43–58.

[4]Judith J. Wurtman, *Managing Your Mind & Mood Through Food* (New York: Harper and Row, 1986).

[5] Chase, 1993.

[6]OSHA Regulations (Standards—29CFR)—1910.95—Occupational noise exposure.

[7]A. Axelsson, A. Eliasson, and B. Israelsson, "Hearing in Pop/Rock Musicians: A Follow-Up Study," *Ear Hear* 16/3 (1995): 245–53.

R. Hétu and M. Fortin, "Potential Risk of Hearing Damage Associated with Exposure to Highly Amplified Music," *Journal of the American Academy of Audiology* 6/5 (1995): 378–86.

T. W. Wong, C. A. Van Hasselt, L. S. Tang, and P. C. Yiu, "The Use of Personal Cassette Players Among Youths and Its Effects on Hearing," *Public Health* 104/5 (1990): 327–30.

[8]Furman, 1978.

Smith and Morris, 1976.

[9]Brown and Mankowski, 1993.

[10]Amy Beckett, "The Effects of Music on Exercise as Determined by Physiological Recovery Heart Rates and Distance," *Journal of Music Therapy* 27/3 (1990): 126–36.

[11]Steve Wulf, "Double Fast," *Time* 8/12/96: 44–47.

[12]Smith and Morris, 1976, 1977.

[13]Kathleen Kelleher, "The Sleepless Society," *The Los Angeles Times* 4/29/96: E1+.

[14]Chase, 1993.

[15]J. Ghika, M. Tennis, J. Growdon, E. Hoffman, and K. Johnson, "Environment-Driven Responses in Progressive Supranuclear Palsy," *Journal of Neurological Science* 130/1 (1995): 104–11.

[16]Oliver Sacks, *Awakenings* (New York: E. P. Dutton, 1983).

[17] Epstein, 1995.

[18] Jourdain, 1997.

[19]Beckett, 1990.

[20]N. Becker, S. Brett, C. Chambliss, K. Crowers, P. Haring, C. Marsh, and R. Montemayor, "Mellow and Frenetic Antecedent Music During Athletic Performance of Children, Adults, and Seniors," *Perceptual and Motor Skills* 79/2 (1994): 1043–46.

K. A. Brownley, R. G. McMurray, and A. C. Hackney, "Effects of Music on Physiological and Affective Responses to Graded Treadmill Exercise in

Trained and Untrained Runners," *International Journal of Psychophysiology* 19/3 (1995): 193–201.

[21]K. M. Hume and J. Crossman, "Musical Reinforcement of Practice Behaviors Among Competitive Swimmers," *Journal of Applied Behavior Analysis* 25/3 (1992): 665–70.

[22]M. A. Thornby, F. Haas, and K. Axen, "Effect of Distractive Auditory Stimuli on Exercise Tolerance in Patients with COPD," *Chest* 107/5 (1995): 1213–17.

[23]Kate Gfeller, "Musical Components and Styles Preferred By Young Adults for Aerobic Fitness Activities," *Journal of Music Therapy* 25/1 (1988): 28–43.

[24]M. Vittitow, I. M. Windmill, J. W. Yates, and D. R. Cunningham, "Effect of Simultaneous Exercise and Noise Exposure (Music) on Hearing," *Journal of the American Academy of Audiology* 5/5 (1994): 343–48.

[25]Steve Wagge, personal communication, 12/28/96.

[26]Beckett, 1990.

[27]Beckett, 1990.

VanderArk and Ely, 1993.

[28]John M. Geringer and Clifford K. Madsen, "Tuning Preferences in Recorded Popular Music," *Applications of Research in Music Behavior*, Clifford K. Madsen and Carol A. Prickett, eds. (Tuscaloosa and London: The University of Alabama Press, 1987): 204–12.

[29]Thaut, Schleiffers, and Davis, 1991.

[30]F. L. Mertesdorf, "Cycle Exercising in Time with Music," *Perceptual and Motor Skills* 78/3 (1994): 123–41.

[31]Avram Goldstein, "Thrills in Response to Music and Other Stimuli," *Physiological Psychology* 8/1 (1980): 126–29.

[32] Jourdain, 1997.

[33] Storr, 1992.

[34]Leonard B. Meyer, *Emotion and Meaning In Music* (Chicago: University of Chicago Press, 1956).

[35]M. A. Wallach, "Two Correlates of Symbolic Sexual Arousal: Level of Anxiety and Liking for Esthetic Material," *Journal of Abnormal and Social Psychology* 61 (1960): 396–401.

[36]K. Blum, P. J. Sheridan, R. C. Wood, E. R. Braverman, T. J. Chen, and D. E. Comings, "Dopamine D2 Receptor Gene Variants: Association and Linkage Studies in Impulsive-Addictive-Compulsive Behaviour," *Pharmacogenetics* 5/3 (1995): 121–41.

B. Castellani and L. Rugle, "A Comparison of Pathological Gamblers to Alcoholics and Cocaine Misusers on Impulsivity, Sensation Seeking, and Craving," *International Journal of the Addictions* 30/3 (1995): 275–89.

S. Hamagaki, "The Dialectic of the Obsessionality and the Dissociativity: Toward a Psycho-Pathology of Binge-Eating," *Seishin Shinkeigaku Zasshi* 97/1 (1995): 1–30.

S. Herpertz, "Self-Injurious Behaviour: Psychopathological and Nosological Characteristics in Subtypes of Self-Injurers," *Acta Psychiatrica Scandinavica* 91/1 (1995): 57–68.

S. Herpertz, S. M. Steinmeyer, D. Marx, A. Oidtmann, and H. Sass, "The Significance of Aggression and Impulsivity for Self-Mutilative Behavior," *Pharmacopsychiatry* 28/2 Suppl. (1995): 64–72.

W. H. Kaye, A. M. Bastiani, and H. Moss, "Cognitive Style of Patients with Anorexia Nervosa and Bulimia Nervosa," *International Journal of Eating Disorders* 18/3 (1995): 287–90.

S. L. McElroy, P. E. Keck, Jr., and K. A. Phillips, "Kleptomania, Compulsive Buying, and Binge Eating Disorder," *Journal of Clinical Psychiatry* 56/4 Suppl (1995): 14–26.

[37]Edwin Atlee, *An Inaugural Essay on the Influence of Music in the Cure of Diseases* (Philadelphia: B. Graves, 1804).

[38]Susan McClary, *Feminine Endings: Music, Gender, and Sexuality* (Minneapolis: University of Minnesota Press, 1991).

[39]These characteristics of Energizing music are drawn from the following research. E. T. Gaston, "Dynamic Music Factors in Mood Change," *Music Educators Journal* 37 (1951): 42–44.

J. A. Prögler, "Searching for Swing: Participatory Discrepancies in the Jazz Rhythm Section," *Ethnomusicology* 39/1 (1995): 21–54.

Smith and Morris, 1976, 1977.

[40]McLaughlin, 1970.

Chapter Two

[1] Cohen and Granot, 1992.

Gail C. Mornhinweg, "Effects of Music Preference and Selection on Stress Reduction," *Journal of Holistic Nursing* 10/2 (1992): 101–09.

Peretti and Swenson, 1974.

P. O. Peretti, "Changes in Galvanic Skin Response as Affected by Musical Selection, Sex, and Academic Discipline," *Journal of Psychology* 89 (1975): 183–87.

Liesl-Vivoni Ramos, "The Effects of On-Hold Telephone Music on the Number of Premature Connections to a Statewide Protective Services Abuse Hot Line," *Journal of Music Therapy* 30/2 (1993): 199–229.

Smith and Morris, 1976, 1977.

Michael H. Thaut and William B. Davis, "The Influence of Subject-Selected versus Experimenter-Chosen Music on Affect, Anxiety, and Relaxation," *Journal of Music Therapy* 30/4 (1993): 210–33.

VanderArk and Ely, 1992.

[2] B. Blumenstein, I. Breslav, M. Bar-Eli, G. Tenenbaum, and Y. Weinstein, "Regulation of Mental States and Biofeedback Techniques: Effects on Breathing Pattern," *Biofeedback and Self Regulation* 20/2 (1995): 169–83.

Davis and Thaut, 1989.

C. Edwards, C. Eagle, J. Pennebaker, and T. Tunks. "Relationships Among Elements of Music and Physiological Responses of Listeners," *Applications of Music in Medicine*, C. D. Maranto, ed. (Washington, DC: National Association for Music Therapy, 1991): 41–47.

P. M. Lehrer, S. M. Hochron, T. Mayne, S. Isenberg, V. Carlson, A. M. Lasoski, J. Gilchrist, D. Morales, and L. Rausch, "Relaxation and Music Therapies for Asthma Among Patients Prestabilized on Asthma Medicine," *Journal of Behavioral Medicine* 17/1 (1994): 1–24.

Mornhinweg, 1992.

Peretti, 1975.

H. Sakamoto, S. Suguira, F. Hayashi, and C. Inagaki, "Individual Differences in Image and Pulse-Wave Responses Elicited by Listening to Music," *Nippon Eiseigaku Zasshi* 45/6 (1991): 1053–60.

Jayne M. Standley, "The Effect of Vibrotactile and Auditory Stimuli on Perception of Comfort, Heart Rate, and Peripheral Finger Temperature," *Journal of Music Therapy* 28/3 (1991): 120–34.

[3] Katy A. Pearce, "Effects of Different Types of Music on Physical Strength," *Perceptual and Motor Skills* 53/2 (1981): 351–52.

[4] M. Möckler, T. Störk, J. Vollert, L Röcker, O. Danne, H. Hochrein, H. Eichstädt, U. Frei, "Stress Reduction Through Listening to Music: Effect on Stress Hormones, Hemodynamics and Mental State in Patients with Arterial Hypertension and in Healthy Persons," *Deutsch Medizinische Wochenschrift* 120/21 (1995): 745–52.

VanderArk and Ely, 1992.

[5] K. Allen and J. Blascovich, "Effects of Music on Cardiovascular Reactivity Among Surgeons," *Journal of the American Medical Association* 272/11 (1994): 882–84.

J. E. Borling, "The Effect of Sedative Music on Alpha Rhythm and Focused Attention in High-Creative and Low-Creative Subjects," *Journal of Music Therapy* 18/2 (1981): 101–08.

Blumenstein et al., 1995.

Davis and Thaut, 1989.

M. Kabuto, T. Kageyama, and H. Nitta, "EEG Power Spectrum Changes Due to Listening to Pleasant Music and Their Relation to Relaxation Effects," *Nippon Eiseigaku Zasshi* 48/4 (1993): 807–18.

Gaston, 1951.

Kabuto et al., 1993.

Lehrer et al., 1994.

Sammi Liebman and Aileen MacLaren, "The Effects of Music and Relaxation on Third Trimester Anxiety in Adolescent Pregnancy," *Journal of Music Therapy* 28/2 (1991): 89–100.

Peretti and Swenson, 1974.

Sheri L. Robb, Ray J. Nichols, Randi L. Rutan, Bonnie L. Bishop, and Jayne C. Parker, "The Effects of Music Assisted Relaxation on Preoperative Anxiety," *Journal of Music Therapy* 32/1 (1995): 2–21.

Smith and Morris, 1976, 1977.

Standley, 1991.

Thaut and Davis, 1993.

White, J. M. "Music Therapy: An Intervention to Reduce Anxiety in the Myocardial Infarction Patient." *Clinical Nurse Specialist* 6/2 (1992): 58–63.

M. J. Winter, S. Paskin, and T. Baker, "Music Reduces Stress and Anxiety in Patients in the Surgical Holding Area," *Journal of Post Anesthetic Nursing* 9/6 (1994): 340–43.

[6]R. S. Lazarus, *Psychological Stress and the Coping Process* (New York: Springer-Verlag, 1966).

C. D. Spielberger, *Manual for the State-Trait Anxiety Inventory* (Palo Alto, CA: Consulting Psychologists Press, 1983).

[7]Mornhinweg, 1992.

[8]Thomas F. Gordon and Paul D'Angelo, "Conceptualizing 'Familiarity' in Music Listening: Implications for Health Research," paper presented at the Annual Conference of the Society for Music Perception and Cognition, Philadelphia, Pa., 1993.

[9]Altschuler, 1948.

Gatewood, 1921.

Mathews, 1806.

Shatin, 1970.

[10]Allison, 1992.

Lehrer et al., 1994.

[11]M. Fredrickson and R. Gunnarson, "Psychobiology of Stage Fright: The Effect of Public Performance on Neuroendocrine, Cardiovascular and Subjective Reactions," *Biological Psychology* 33/1 (1992): 51–61.

[12]Möckler, Störk, Vollert, Röcker, Danne, Hochrein, Eichstädt, and Frei, 1995.

[13]Smith and Morris, 1977.

[14]Valerie N. Stratton, "Influence of Music and Socializing on Perceived Stress While Waiting," *Perceptual and Motor Skills* 75/1 (1992): 334.

[15]J. C. Chebat, C. Gelinas-Chebat, and P. Filiatrault, "Interactive Effects of Musical and Visual Cues on Time Perception: An Application to Waiting Lines in Banks," *Perceptual and Motor Skills* 77/3 (1993): 995–1020.

Ramos, 1993.

Stratton, 1992.

[16]T. Ikeda, "Concentration-Effect and Underestimation of Time by Acoustic Stimuli," *Shinrigaku Kankyu (Japanese Journal of Psychology)* 63/3 (1992): 157–62.

[17]Paul Dean, "On the Cruel Freeways, It's Don't Get Mad—Get Creative," *Los Angeles Times* 11/13/96: E1+.

[18]D. J. Blood and S. J. Ferriss, "Effects of Background Music on Anxiety, Satisfaction with Communication, and Productivity," *Psychological Reports* 72/1 (1993):171–77.

A. R. Peden, "Music: Making the Connection with People Who Are Homeless," *Journal of Psychological Nursing and Mental Health Services* 31/7 (1993): 17–20.

Ramos, 1993.

Smith and Morris, 1977.

W. Tang, X. Yao, and Z. Zheng, "Rehabilitative Effect of Music Therapy for Residual Schizophrenia: A One-Month Randomized Controlled Trial in Shanghai," *British Journal of Psychiatry Supplement* 24 (1994): 38–44.

[19]Bruce A. Prueter and Joseph Mezzano, "Effects of Background Music upon Initial Counseling Interaction," *Journal of Music Therapy* 10 (1973): 205–12.

[20]Michael H. Thaut, "The Influence of Music Therapy Interventions on Self-Rated Changes in Relaxation, Affect, and Thought in Psychiatric Prisoner-Patients," *Journal of Music Therapy* 26/3 (1989): 155–66.

[21]Blood and Ferriss, 1993.

Clarke S. Harris, Richard J. Bradley, and Sharon K. Titus, "A Comparison of the Effects of Hard Rock and Easy Listening on the Frequency of Observed Inappropriate Behaviors: Control of Environmental Antecedents in a Large Public Area," *Journal of Music Therapy* 29/1 (1992): 6–17.

[22]American Psychological Association, "Answers to Your Questions About Panic Disorder," Washington, DC, nd.

[23]G. H. Eifert, L. Craill, E. Carey, and C. O'Connor, "Affect Modification Through Evaluative Conditioning with Music," *Behavior Research and Therapy* 26 (1988): 321–30.

[24]S. F. Kelly, "The Use of Music as Hypnotic Suggestion," *American Journal of Clinical Hypnosis* 36/2 (1993): 83–90.

[25]Joachim-Ernst Berendt, *The World Is Sound–Nada Brahma* (Rochester, VT: Destiny Books, 1987).

[26]Borling, 1981.

Furman, 1978.

[27]Petsche, 1992a and 1992b.

[28]Cohen and Granot, 1992.

Hough, Daniel, Snow, O'Brien, and Hume, 1994.

Nowak, 1995.

Schlaug, Jäncke, Huang, and Steinmetz, 1993, 1995.

[29]Diana Spies Pope, "Music, Noise and the Human Voice in the Nurse-Patient Environment," *Image—The Journal of Nursing Scholarship* 27/4 (1995): 291–96.

J. M. Standley and C. K. Madsen, "Comparison of Infant Preferences and Responses to Auditory Stimuli: Music, Mother, and Other Female Voice," *Journal of Music Therapy* 27/2 (1990): 54–97.

[30]G. C. Mornhinweg and R. R. Voignier, "Music for Sleep Disturbance in the Elderly," *Journal of Holistic Nursing* 13/3 (1995): 248–54.

[31]Columbia University Health Service, "While You Weren't Sleeping," *Healthwise Highlights* 4/1 (1995).

Kelleher, 1996.

[32]These characteristics of Relaxing music are drawn from the research cited in notes 1 through 5.

[33]Davis and Thaut, 1989.

Thaut and Davis, 1993.

[34]Steven Halpern with Louis Savary, *Sound Health: The Music and Sounds That Make Us Whole* (San Francisco: Harper & Row, 1985): 30.

[35]Ramos 1993.

[36]S. Ogata, "Human EEG Responses to Classical Music and Simulated White Noise: Effects of a Musical Loudness Component on Consciousness," *Perceptual and Motor Skills* 80/3 (1995): 779–90.

[37]C. W. Mitchell, "Effects of Subliminally Presented Auditory Suggestions of Itching on Scratching Behavior," *Perceptual and Motor Skills* 80/1 (1995): 87–96.

Myra J. Staum and Melissa Brotons, "The Influence of Auditory Subliminals on Behavior: A Series of Investigations," *Journal of Music Therapy* 29/3 (1992): 130–185.

[38]S. E. Trehub, A. M Unyk, and L. J. Trainor, "Adults Identify Infant-Directed Music Across Cultures," *Infant Behavior and Development* 16/2 (1993): 193–211.

Chapter Three

[1]Holden, 1994.

Hotz, 1993.

Rauscher, Shaw, and Ky, 1993.

[2] Jourdain, 1997.

[3]C. B. Carstens, E. Huskins, and G. W. Hounshell, "Listening to Mozart May Not Enhance Performance on the Revised Minnesota Paper Form Board Test," *Psychological Reports* 77/1 (1995): 111–14.

[4]Rauscher et al., 1994, 1995.

[5]M. Hassler, N. Birbaumer, and A. Feil, "Musical Talent and Visual-Spatial Abilities: A Longitudinal Study," *Psychology of Music* 13/2 (1985): 99–113.

[6]Hassler, Birbaumer, and Feil, 1985.

[7]Leng and Shaw, 1991.

Leng and Shaw, "Toward a Neural Theory of Higher Brain Function Using Music as a Window," paper presented at the Second International Conference on Music Perception and Cognition, UCLA, Los Angeles, CA, 1992.

[8]Rauscher, Shaw, and Ky, 1995.

Rauscher, Shaw, Levine, Ky, and Wright, 1994.

Frances H. Rauscher, Gordon L. Shaw, Linda J. Levine, and Eric L. Wright, "Pilot Study Indicates Music Training of Three-Year-Olds Enhances Specific Spatial Reasoning Skills," paper presented at the Economic Summit of the National Association of Music Merchants, Newport Beach, CA, 1993.

[9]Frances H. Rauscher, Gordon L. Shaw, Linda J. Levine, Eric L. Wright, Wendy R. Dennis, and Robert L. Newcomb. "Music Improves Reasoning in Preschool Children." *Neurological Research* 19 (February 1997): 2–8.

[10]Valerie N. Stratton and Annette H. Zalanowski, "The Effects of Music and Cognition on Mood," *Psychology of Music* 19 (1991): 121–27.

[11]Leon K. Miller and Michael Schyb, "Facilitation and Interference by Background Music," *Journal of Music Therapy* 26/1 (1989): 42–54.

[12]T. Taniguchi, "Mood Congruent Effects by Music on Word Cognition," *Shinrigaku Kenkyu (Japanese Journal of Psychology)* 62/2 (1991): 88–95.

Michael Thaut and Shannon K. de l'Etoile, "The Effects of Music on Mood State–Dependent Recall," *Journal of Music Therapy* 30/2 (1993): 70–80.

[13]L. L. Morton, J. R. Kershner, and L. S. Siegel, "The Potential for Therapeutic Applications of Music on Problems Related to Memory and Attention," *Journal of Music Therapy* 27/4 (1990): 195–208.

[14]Kate Gfeller, "Musical Mnemonics as an Aid to Retention with Normal and Learning Disabled Students," *Journal of Music Therapy* 20 (1983): 179–89.

[15]Sheila Ostrander and Lynn Schroeder, with Nancy Ostrander, *Superlearning 2000* (New York: Delacorte Press, 1994).

Colin Rose, *Accelerated Learning* (New York: Dell Books, 1989).

[16]S. A. Henry and R. G. Swartz, "Enhancing Healthcare Education with Accelerated Learning Techniques," *Journal of Nursing Staff Development* 11/1 (1995): 21–24.

J. Hoffman, S. Summers, J. A. Neff, S. Hanson, and K. Pierce, "The Effects of 60 Beats per Minute Music on Test Taking Anxiety Among Nursing Students," *Journal of Nursing Education* 29/2 (1990): 66–70.

[17]J. Cartwright and G. Huckaby, "Intensive Preschool Language Program," *Journal of Music Therapy* 9/3 (1972): 147–55.

Cynthia M. Colwell, "Therapeutic Applications of Music in the Whole Language Kindergarten," *Journal of Music Therapy* 31/4 (1994): 238–47.

Lori A. Fitzgerald, "A Musical Approach for Teaching English Reading to Limited English Speakers," master's thesis, National-Louis University, 1994.

H. Gingold and E. Abravanel, "Music as a Mnemonic: The Effects of Good and Bad Music Settings on Verbatim Recall of Short Passages by Young Children," *Psychomusicology* 7/1 (1987): 25–39.

C. K. Madsen, C. H. Madsen, Jr. and D. E. Michel, "The Use of Music Stimuli in Teaching Language Discrimination," *Research in Music Behavior*, C. K. Madsen, R. D. Greer, and C. H. Madsen, Jr., eds. (New York: Teachers College Press, 1975).

Sitka A. Madsen, "The Effect of Music Paired With and Without Gestures on the Learning and Transfer of New Vocabulary: Experimenter-Derived Nonsense Words," *Journal of Music Therapy* 28/4 (1991): 222–30.

W. Sims, "Effects of Pitch and Rhythm on the Short-Term Memorization of Nonsense Syllable Sequences by College Students," *Contributions to Music Education* 8 (1980): 73–91.

David E. Wolfe and Candice Hom, "Use of Melodies as Structural Prompts for Learning and Retention of Sequential Verbal Information by Preschool Students," *Journal of Music Therapy* 30/2 (1993): 100–18.

[18]George List, "Speech Melody and Song Melody in Central Thailand," *Intonation*, D. Bolinger, ed. (Baltimore: Penguin Books, 1972) 263–81.

[19]Gerard Alberic, "En Chanson: 'Pourquoi' et 'Comment,' " *Francais dans le Monde* 263 (1994): 111–16.

Myra L. Staum, "Music as an Intonational Cue for Bilingual Language Acquisition," *Applications of Research in Music Behavior*, Clifford K. Madsen and Carol A. Prickett, eds. (Tuscaloosa and London: The University of Alabama Press, 1987), 285–96.

[20]C. Etaugh and P. Ptasnik, "Effects of Studying to Music and Poststudy Relaxation on Reading Comprehension," *Perceptual and Motor Skills* 55/1 (1982): 141–42.

C. N. Mulliken and W. A. Henk, "Using Music as a Background for Reading: An Exploratory Study," *Journal of Reading* 28/4 (1985): 353–58.

[21]Etaugh and Ptasnik, 1982.

[22]Tharyll W. Morrow-Pretlow, "Using Rap Lyrics to Encourage At-Risk Elementary Grade Urban Learners to Read for Pleasure," Ed.D. Practicum, Nova Southeastern University, 1994.

[23]Miller and Schyb, 1989.

Mariko Osaka and Naoyuki Osaka, "Effect of Musical Tempo Upon Reading Performance," paper presented at the Second International Conference on Music Perception and Cognition, Los Angeles, CA, 1992.

[24]Irene Berkowitz, "Effects of Background Music on Reading Comprehension: Performance Enhancement or Deterioration," paper presented at the Annual Conference of the Society for Music Perception and Cognition, Philadelphia, PA, 1993.

Miller and Schyb, 1989.

[25]Beth Landis and Polly Carder, *The Eclectic Curriculum in American Music Education: Contributions of Dalcroze, Kodaly and Orff* (Reston, VA: Music Educators National Conference, 1972).

[26]Henry Barnes, *An Introduction to Waldorf Education* (Chestnut Ridge, NY: Mercury Press, 1985).

[27]Don G. Campbell, *Introduction to the Musical Brain* (St. Louis, MO: MMB Music, 1986).

[28]Schlaug, Jäncke, Huang, Staiger, and Steinmetz, 1995.

[29]T. Elbert, C. Pantev, C. Weinbruch, B. Rockstroh, and E. Taub, "Increased Cortical Representation of the Fingers of the Left Hand in String Players," *Science* 270/5234 (1995): 305–07.

[30] Johnson, Petsche, Richter, von Stein, and Filz, "The Dependence of Coherence Estimates of Spontaneous EEG on Gender and Music Training," *Music Perception* 13 (1996): 563–82.

[31]Martin F. Gardiner, Alan Fox, Faith Knowles, Donna Jeffrey, "Learning Improved by Arts Training," *Nature* 381 (1996): 284.

[32]Blakeslee, 1995.

Holden, 1994.

Rauscher, Shaw, Levine, and Wright, 1993.

Rauscher et al., 1994.

Rauscher, Shaw, Levine, Wright, Dennis, and Newcomb, 1997.

[33]Leng and Shaw, 1992.

[34]W. Kessen, J. Levine, and K. A. Wendrich, "The Imitation of Pitch in Infants," *Infant Behavior and Development* 2 (1979): 931–99.

[35]Marcel R. Zentner and Jerome Kagan, "Perception of Music by Infants," *Nature* 383/6595 (1996): 29.

M. P. Lynch, L. B. Short, and R. Chua, "Contributions of Experience to the Development of Musical Processing in Infancy," *Developmental Psychobiology* 28/7 (1995): 377–98.

[36]Jill Jarnow, *All Ears: How to Choose and Use Recorded Music for Children* (New York: Viking, 1991).

[37]Miller and Schyb, 1989.

[38]Thaut and de l'Etoile, 1993.

[39]Ostrander and Schroeder, 1994.

[40] Jarnow, 1991.

Arlette Zenatti, "Children's Musical Cognition and Taste," *Psychology and Music: The Understanding of Melody and Rhythm*, Thomas J. Tighe and W. Jay Dowling, eds. (Hillsdale, NJ: Lawrence Erlbaum Associates, 1993): 177–96.

[41]Jarnow, 1991.

[42] Zenatti, 1993.

[43] Fred H. Gage. "More Hippocampal Neurons in Adult Mice Living in an Enriched Environment," *Nature* 386/6624 (1997): 493–95.

[44]F. A. Albersnagel, "Velten and Musical Mood Induction Procedures: A Comparison with Accessibility of Thought Associations," *Behavior Research and Therapy* 26/1 (1988): 79–86.

Eileen Gail Nix, "The Relationships Among Classical Background Music, Time-on-Task Behavior, and Academic Achievement of Sixth-Grade Students," doctoral dissertation, University of Georgia, 1991.

[45]Borling, 1981.

Furman, 1978.

[46]Miller and Schyb, 1989.

[47]Morton, Kershner, and Siegel, 1990.

Osaka and Osaka, 1992.

Thaut and de l'Etoile, 1993.

[48] Blood and Ferriss, 1993.

Smith and Morris, 1977.

[49]Allen and Blascovich, 1994.

[50]Borling, 1981.

[51]Miller and Schyb, 1989.

[52]Furman, 1978.

[53]Osaka and Osaka, 1992.

[54]Morton, Kershner, and Siegel, 1990.

Thaut and de l'Etoile, 1993.

[55]Barnes, 1988.

[56]Clifford K. Madsen, "Background Music: Competiton for Focus of Attention," *Applications of Research in Music Behavior*, Clifford K. Madsen and Carol A. Prickett, eds. (Tuscaloosa and London: The University of Alabama Press, 1987), 315–25.

[57]Borling, 1981.

[58]Barnes, Stephen H., *Muzak: The Hidden Messages in Music* (Lewiston/ Queenstown: The Edwin Mellen Press, 1988).

[59]David Huron, "The Ramp Archetype and the Maintenance of Passive Auditory Attention," *Music Perception* 10/1 (1992): 83–91.

[60]Morton, Kershner, and Seigel, 1990.

[61]R. D. Greer, "An Operant Approach to Motivation and Affect: Ten Years of Research in Music Learning," *Ann Arbor Symposium* (Reston, VA: Music Educators National Conference, 1980).

Hume and Crossman, 1992.

Gladys Williams and Laura G. Dorow, "Changes in Complaints and Non-Complaints of a Chronically Depressed Psychiatric Patient as a Function of an Interrupted Music/Verbal Feedback Package," *Journal of Music Therapy* 20/3 (1983): 143–55.

C. W. Wilson and B. L. Hopkins, "The Effects of Contingent Music on the Intensity of Noise in Junior High Economics Classes," *Journal of Applied Behavior Analysis* 6 (1973): 269–75.

[62]These characteristics of Focusing music are drawn from the following research:

Allen and Blascovich, 1994.

Blood and Ferriss, 1993.

Borling, 1981.

Jourdain, 1997.

Miller and Schyb, 1989.

Morton et al., 1990.

Ostrander and Schroeder, 1994.

Smith and Morris, 1977.

Thaut and de l'Etoile, 1993.

Chapter Four

[1]Spies and Pope, 1995.

[2]Standley, 1986.

[3]W. Andritzy, "Medical Students and Alternative Medicine—A Survey," *Gesundheitswesen* 57/6 (1995): 345–48.

[4]J. Escher, U. Hohmann, and C. Wasem, "Music Therapy and Internal Medicine," *Schweizerische Rundschau fur Medizin Praxis* 82/36 (1993): 957–63.

[5]G. J. Daniels and P. McCabe, "Nursing Diagnosis and Natural Therapies: A Symbiotic Relationship," *Journal of Holistic Nursing* 12/2 (1994): 184–92.

[6]Atlee, 1804.

Mathews, 1806.

Podolsky, 1939.

Schullian and Schoer, 1948.

[7]Marina Roseman, "Healing Sounds from the Malaysian Rainforest: Temiar Music and Medicine," *Comparative Studies of Health Systems and Medical Care, Vol. 28* (University of California Press, 1991).

[8]Bruno Deschênes, "Healing Beyond Music," paper presented at the Fifth International Conference on the Study of Shamanism and Alternate Modes of Healing, San Rafael, CA, 1988.

Kay Gardner, *Sounding the Inner Landscape: Music as Medicine* (Stonington, ME: Caduceus Publications, 1990).

Halpern and Savary, 1985.

[9]D. Elliott, "A Review of Nursing Strategies to Reduce Patient Anxiety in Coronary Care, Part 2," *Australian Critical Care* 5/3 (1992): 10–16.

Escher et al., 1993.

G. C. Morhinweg and R. R. Voignier, "Holistic Nursing Interventions," *Orthopedic Nursing* 14/4 (1995): 20–24.

[10]Dale Anderson, *The Orchestra Conductor's Secret to Health and Long Life* (Chronimed, 1997).

[11] Rider, Floyd, and Kirkpatrick, 1985.

[12] Dale Bartlett, Donald Kaufman, and Roger Smeltekop, "The Effects of Music Listening and Perceived Sensory Experiences on the Immune System as Measured by Interleukin-1 and Cortisol," *Journal of Music Therapy* 30/4 (1993): 194–209.

[13]Möckler, Störk, Vollert, Röcker, Danne, Hochrein, Eichstädt, Frei, 1995.

[14]Marina Roseman, "The Pragmatics of Aesthetics: The Performance of Healing among Senoi Temiar," *Social Science and Medicine* 27/8 (1988): 811–18.

Roseman, 1991.

[15]J. Hoskins, "The Drum Is the Shaman, the Spear Guides His Voice," *Social Science and Medicine* 27/8 (1988): 819–28.

[16]Rider, et al., 1985.

[17]Davis and Thaut, 1989.

Harrer and Harrer, 1977.

Updike, 1990.

VanderArk and Ely, 1992.

VanderArk and Ely, 1993.

Wheeler, 1985.

[18]L. Epstein, M. Hersen, and D. Hemphill, "Music Feedback in the Treatment of Tension Headache: An Experimental Case Study," *Journal of Behavior Therapy and Experimental Psychology* 5 (1974): 59–63.

[19]Lehrer, Hochron, Mayne, Isenberg, Carlson, Lasoski, Gilchrist, Morales, and Rausch, 1994.

[20]Standley, 1986.

[21]C. Ishii, S. Hagihara, and R. Minamisawa, "Effects of Music on Relieving Pain Associated with a Compulsory Posture," *Nihon Kango Kagakkai (Journal of Japan Academy of Nursing Science)* 13/1 (1993): 20–27.

[22]Florence Nightingale, *Notes on Nursing: What It Is and What It Is Not* (Philadelphia: J. B. Lippincott, 1992, orig. 1859).

[23]Pope, 1995.

[24]J. P. Griffin, "The Impact of Noise on Critically Ill People," *Holistic Nursing Practice* 6/4 (1992): 53–66.

[25]D. O. McCarthy, M. E. Ouimet, and J. M. Daun, "Shades of Florence Nightingale: Potential Impact of Noise Stress on Wound Healing," *Holistic Nursing Practice* 5/4 (1991): 39–48.

[26] White, 1992.

[27]C. A. L. Bolwerk, "Effects of Relaxing Music on State Anxiety in Myocardial Infarction Patients," *Critical Care Nursing Quarterly* 13/2 (1990): 63–72.

Helen L. Bonny, "Music Listening for Intensive Coronary Care Units: A Pilot Project," *Journal of Music Therapy* 3/1 (1983): 4–16.

[28]Updike, 1990.

[29]D. K. Fontaine, "Nonpharmacologic Management of Patient Distress During Mechanical Ventilation," *Critical Care Clinics* 10/4 (1994): 695–708.

[30]L. L. Chlan, "Psychophysiologic Responses of Mechanically Ventilated

Patients to Music: A Pilot Study," *American Journal of Critical Care* 4/3 (1995): 233–38.

[31]Standley, 1986.

[32]David Aldridge, "Music Therapy in Intensive Care," *The Arts in Psychotherapy* 18 (1991): 359–62.

[33]M. J. Staum, "Music and Rhythmic Stimuli in the Rehabilitation of Gait Disorders," *Journal of Music Therapy* 20 (1983): 69–87.

[34]Thornby, Haas, and Axen, 1995.

[35]M. E. Boyle, Operant Procedures and the Comatose Patient, doctoral dissertation, Teachers College, Columbia University, 1981.

[36]Standley, 1986.

[37]Cynthia Allison Davis, "The Effects of Music and Basic Relaxation Instruction on Pain and Anxiety of Women Undergoing In-Office Gynecological Procedures," *Journal of Music Therapy* 24/4 (1992): 202–16.

[38]Davis, 1992.

L. Magill-Levreault, "Music Therapy in Pain and Symptom Management," *Journal of Palliative Care* 1/4 (1993): 42–48.

M. McCaffery, "Nursing Approaches to Nonpharmacological Pain Control," *International Journal of Nursing Studies* 27/1 (1990): 1–5.

Standley, 1986.

B. Whipple and N. J. Glynn, "Quantification of the Effects of Listening to Music as a Noninvasive Method of Pain Control," *Scholarly Inquiry for Nursing Practice* 6/1 (1992): 43–62.

[39]Monte S. Buchsbaum, Robert Lavine, and Mark Poncy, "Auditory Analgesia: Somatosensory Evoked Response and Subjective Pain Rating," *Psychophysiology* 13 (1976): 140–48.

[40]H. Cherry and I. Pallin, "Music as a Supplement in Nitrous Oxide Oxygen Anesthesia," *Anesthesiology* 9 (1948): 391–99.

[41]R. A. Atterbury, "Auditory Pre-Sedation for Oral Surgery Patients," *Audioanalgesia* 38/6 (1974): 12–14.

W. J. Gardner and J. C. Licklider, "Auditory Analgesia in Dental Operation," *Journal of the American Dental Association* 59 (1959): 1144–50.

W. Gardner, J. C. R. Licklider, and A. Z. Weisz, "Suppression of Pain by Sound," *Science* 132 (1960): 32–33.

H. L. Jacobson, "The Effect of Sedative Music on the Tensions, Anxiety and Pain Experienced by Mental Patients During Dental Procedures," *Music Therapy 1956: Book of Proceedings of the National Association for Music Therapy, Inc.,* E. T. Gaston, ed. (Lawrence, KS: National Association for Music Therapy, Inc.): 231–34.

L. Long and J. Johnson, "Dental Practice Using Music to Aid Relaxation and Relieve Pain," *Dental Survey* 54 (1978): 35–38.

H. L. Monsey, "Preliminary Report of the Clinical Efficacy of Audioanalgesia," *Journal of California State Dental Association* 36 (1960): 432–37.

T. Oyama, K. Hatano, Y. Sato, M. Kudo, R. Spintge, and R. Droh, "Endocrine Effect of Anxiolytic Music in Dental Patients," *Angst, Schmerz, Musik in der Anasthesie*, R. Droh and R. Spintge, eds. (Basel: Editions Roche, 1983): 143–46.

R. Schermer, "Distraction Analgesia Using the Stereogesic Portable," *Military Medicine* 125 (1960): 67–78.

Standley, 1986.

Standley, 1991.

R. L. Weisbrod, "Audio Analgesia Revisited," *Anesthesia Progress* (January 1969): 8–15.

[42]J. M. Dubois, T. Bartter, and M. R. Pratter, "Music Improves Patient Comfort Level During Outpatient Bronchoscopy," *Chest* 108/1 (1995): 129–30.

G. Kaempf and M. Amodei, "The Effects of Music on Anxiety," *AORN Journal* 50 (1989): 112–18.

J. J. Menegazzi, P. M. Paris, C. H. Kersteen, B. Flynn, D. E. Trautman, "A Randomized, Controlled Trial of the Use of Music During Laceration Repair," *Annals of Emergency Medicine* 20/4 (1991): 348–50.

K. S. Mowatt, "Background Music During Radiotherapy," *Medical Journal, Australia* 1 (1967): 185–6.

K. C. Palakanis, J. W. DeNobile, W. B. Sweeney, and C. L. Blankenship, "Effect of Music Therapy on State Anxiety in Patients Undergoing Flexible Sigmoidoscopy," *Diseases of the Colon and Rectum* 37/5 (1994): 478–81.

K. J. Slifer, K. Penn-Jones, M. F. Cataldo, R. T. Connor, and E. A. Zerhouni, "Music Enhances Patients' Comfort During MR Imaging," *American Journal of Roentgenology* 156 (1991): 403.

[43]Davis, 1992.

[44]V. I. Rickert, K. J. Kozlowsi, A. M. Warren, A. Hendon, and P. Davis, "Adolescents and Colposcopy: The Use of Different Procedures to Reduce Anxiety," *American Journal of Obstetrics and Gynecology* 170/2 (1994): 504–08.

[45]Davis, 1992.

[46]A. G. Shapiro and H. Cohen, "Auxiliary Pain Relief During Suction Curettage," *Angst, Schmerz, Musik in der Anasthesie,* R. Droh and R. Spintge, eds. (Basel: Editions Roche, 1983) 89–93.

[47]S. L. Beck, "The Therapeutic Use of Music for Cancer-Related Pain," *Oncology Nursing Forum* 18/8 (1991): 1327–37.

G. J. Kerkviet, "Music Therapy May Help Control Cancer Pain," *Journal of the National Cancer Institute* 82/5 (1990): 350–52.

J. A. Schorr, "Music and Pattern Change in Chronic Pain," *ANS Advances in Nursing Science* 15/4 (1993): 27–36.

David E. Wolfe, "Pain Rehabilitation and Music Therapy," *Journal of Music Therapy* 25/4 (1978): 162–78.

[48]E. Christenberry, "The Use of Music Therapy with Burn Patients," *Journal of Music Therapy* 16 (1979): 138–48.

A. C. Miller, L. C. Hickman, and G. K. Lemasters, "A Distraction Technique for Control of Burn Pain," *Journal of Burn Care and Rehabilitation* 13/5 (1992): 576–80.

Standley, 1986.

[49]Christenberry, 1979.

Standley, 1986.

Whipple and Glynn, 1992.

[50]McCaffery, 1990.

Whipple and Glynn, 1992.

[51]Standley, 1986.

[52]Standley, 1986.

[53]B. Miluk-Kolasa, Z. Obminski, R. Stupnicki, and L. Golec, "Effects of Music Treatment on Salivary Cortisol in Patients Exposed to Pre-Surgical Stress," *Experimental and Clinical Endicronology* 102/2 (1994): 118–20.

[54]C. L. Cirina, "Effects of Sedative Music on Patient Preoperative Anxiety," *Today's OR Nurse* 16/3 (1994): 1518.

M. M. Evans and P. A. Rubio, "Music: A Diversionary Therapy," *Today's OR Nurse* 16/4 (1994): 17–22.

V. A. Moss, "Music and the Surgical Patient," *AORN Journal* 48/1 (1988): 64–9.

Robb, Nichols, Rutan, Bishop, and Parker, 1995.

Winter, Paskin, and Baker, 1994.

[55]K. Stevens, "Patients' Perception of Music During Surgery," *Journal of Advanced Nursing* 15/9 (1990): 1045–51.

[56]V. M. Steelman, "Intraoperative Music Therapy," *AORN Journal* 52 (1990): 1026–34.

[57]C. S. Tang, C. J. Ko, S. M. Ng, S. C. Chen, K. I. Cheng, K. L. Yu, and C. K. Tseng, " 'Walkman Music' During Epidural Anesthesia," *Kao-Hsiung i Hsueh Tsa Chih Kaohsiung (Journal of Medical Sciences)* 9/8 (1993): 468–75.

[58]K. Kiviniemi, "Conscious Awareness and Memory During General Anesthesia," *AANA Journal* 62/5 (1994): 441–49.

[59]N. Ochiai, R. Okutani, Y. Yoshimura, and K. Fu, "Perioperative Management of a Patient with Severe Bronchial Asthma Attack," *Masui* 44/8 (1995): 1124–27.

[60]R. G. Locsin, "The Effect of Music on the Pain of Selected Post-Operative Patients," *Journal of Advanced Nursing* 6 (1981): 19–25.

[61]Davis, 1992.

[62]L. Heitz, T. Symreng, and F. L. Scamman, "Effect of Music Therapy in the Postanasthesia Care Unit: A Nursing Intervention," *Journal of Post Anesthesia Nursing* 7/1 (1992): 22–31.

[63]S. Barnason, L. Zimmerman, and J. Nieveen, "The Effects of Music Interventions on Anxiety in the Patient After Coronary Artery Bypass Grafting," *Heart and Lung* 24/2 (1995): 124–32.

[64]M. Good, "A Comparison of the Effects of Jaw Relaxation and Music on Postoperative Pain," *Nursing Research* 44/1: 52–57.

[65]Standley, 1986.

[66] M. E. Clark, R. R. McCorkle, and S. B. Williams, "Music Therapy-Assisted Labor and Delivery," *Journal of Music Therapy* 18/2 (1981): 88–109.

[67]P. A. Codding, "An Exploration of the Uses of Music in the Birthing Process," master's thesis, Florida State University, 1982.

L. Durham and M. Collins, "The Effect of Music as a Conditioning Aid in Prepared Childbirth Education," *Journal of Obstetric, Gynecologic, and Neonatal Nursing* 15/3 (1986): 268–70.

S. B. Hanser, S. C. Larson, and A. S. O'Connell, "The Effect of Music on Relaxation of Expectant Mothers During Labor," *Journal of Music Therapy* 20 (1983): 50–58.

Liebman and MacLaren, 1991.

J. C. Livingston, "Music for the Childbearing Family," *JOGN Nursing* 8/6 (1979): 363–67.

K. M. Stevens, "My Room—Not Theirs! A Case Study of Music During Childbirth," *Journal/ Australian College of Midwives* 5/3 (1992): 27–30.

M. A. Winokur, "The Use of Music as an Audio-Analgesia During Childbirth," master's thesis, Florida State University, 1984.

[68]Standley, 1986.

[69]C. T. Beck, "Postpartum Depressed Mothers' Experiences Interacting with Their Children," *Nursing Research* 45/2 (1996): 98–104.

[70]L. McDonnell, "Paraverbal Therapy in Pediatric Cases with Emotional Complications," *American Journal of Orthopsychiatry* 49/1 (1979): 44–52.

[71]J. Caine, "The Effects of Music on the Selected Stress Behaviors, Weight, Caloric Intake, and Length of Hospital Stay of Premature and Low Birth Weight Neonates in a Newborn Intensive Care Unit," *Journal of Music Therapy* 28/4 (1992): 180–92.

[72]Pope, 1995.

[73]M. Burke, J. Walsh, J. Oehler, and J. Gingras, "Music Therapy Following Suctioning: Four Case Studies," *Neonatal Network* 14/7 (1995): 41–49.

[74] Standley and Madsen, 1990.

[75]J. S. Chapman, "The Relation between Auditory Stimulation of Short Gestation Infants and Their Gross Motor Limb Activity," doctoral dissertation, New York University, 1975.

F. Hicks, "The Role of Music Therapy in the Care of the Newborn," *Nursing Times* 91/38 (1995): 31–33.

Standley, 1986.

[76]J. M. Oehler, "Developmental Care of Low Birth Weight Infants," *Nursing Clinics of North America* 28/2 (1993): 289–301.

[77]T.S. Fagen, "Music Therapy in the Treatment of Anxiety and Fear in Terminal Pediatric Patients," *Music Therapy* 2/1 (1982): 13–23.

L. S. Marley, "The Use of Music with Hospitalized Infants and Toddlers: A Descriptive Study," *Journal of Music Therapy* 21 (1984): 126–32.

L. McDonnell, "Music Therapy with Trauma Patients and Their Families on a Pediatric Service," *Music Therapy* 4/1 (1984): 55–66.

D. Robinson, "Music Therapy in a General Hospital," *Bulletin of the National Association for Music Therapy* 11/3 (1962): 13–18.

[78]S. Fowler-Kerry and J. R. Lander, "Management of Injection Pain in Children," *Pain* 30/2 (1987): 169–75.

[79] Robb, Nichols, Rutan, Bishop, and Parker, 1995.

[80]D. Lane, "Music Therapy: A Gift Beyond Measure," *Oncology Nursing Forum* 19 (1992): 863–67.

[81]V. E. Keller, "Management of Nausea and Vomiting in Children," *Journal of Pediatric Nursing* 10/5 (1995): 280–86.

J. M. Standley and S. B. Hanser, "Music Therapy Research and Applications in Pediatric Oncology Treatment," *Journal of Pediatric Oncology Nursing* 12/1 (1995): 3–8.

M. M. Stevens, L. Dalla Pozza, B. Cavalletto, M. G. Cooper and H. A. Kilham, "Pain and Symptom Control in Pediatric Palliative Care," *Cancer Surveys* 21 (1994): 211–31.

[82]J. Goddaer and I. J. Abraham, "Effects of Relaxing Music on Agitation during Meals among Nursing Home Residents with Severe Cognitive Impairment," *Archives of Psychiatric Nursing* 8/3 (1994): 150–58.

[83]J. A. Casby and M. B. Holm, "The Effect of Music on Repetitive Disruptive Vocalizations of Persons with Dementia," *American Journal of Occupational Therapy* 48/10 (1994): 883–89.

T. R. Lord and J. E. Garner, "Effects of Music on Alzheimer Patients," *Perceptual and Motor Skills* 76/2 (1993): 451–55.

[84]S. Jochims, "Coping with Illness in the Early Phase of Sever Neurologic Diseases: A Contribution of Music Therapy to Psychological Management in Selected Neurologic Disease Pictures," *Psychotherapie, Psychosomatik, Medizinische Psychologie*. 40/3–4 (1990): 115–22.

[85]Tracy Weber, "Tarnishing the Golden Years with Addiction," *Los Angeles Times* 12/20/96: A1+.

[86]X. Chen, "Active Music Therapy for Senile Depression," *Chung-Hua Shen Ching Ching Shen Ko Tsa Chih (Chinese Journal of Neurology and Psychiatry)* 25/4 (1992): 252–53.

Sandra L. Curtis, "The Effect of Music on Pain Relief and Relaxation of the Terminally Ill," *Journal of Music Therapy* 23/1 (1986): 10–24.

A. Deeken, "Death Education as a Way to Improve the Quality of Life of Cancer Patients after a Relapse," *Gan To Kagaku Ryoho* 22/suppl. 1 (1995): 22–25.

Fagen, 1982.

Hanser and Thompson, 1994.

S. Jochims, "Depression in the Elderly; Contribution of Music Therapy to Grief Work," *Zeitschrift fur Gerontologie* 25/6 (1992): 391–96.

[87]T. Schroeder-Shenker, "Music for the Dying: A Personal Account of the New Field of Music-Thanatology—History, Theories, and Clinical Narratives," *Journal of Holistic Nursing* 12/1 (1994): 83–99.

[88]Nightingale, 1992 (1859).

Standley and Madsen, 1990.

Updike, 1990.

[89]Heller, 1987.

Podolsky, 1939.

[90]Livingston, 1979.

Chapter Five

[1]Adaman and Blaney, 1995.

Michael Pignatiello, Cameron J. Camp, S. Thomas Elder, and Lee Anna Rasar, "A Psychophysiological Comparison of the Velten and Musical Mood Induction Techniques," *Journal of Music Therapy* 26/3 (1989): 140–54.

K. Spies, F. W. Hesse, A. Gerrads-Hesse, E. Ueffing, "Experimental Induction of Mood States—Does Addition of Music Improve Self-Disclosure?" *Zeitschrift fur Experimentelle und Angewandte Psychologie* 38/2 (1991): 321–42.

Mark Meirum Tergwot and Flora van Grinsven, "Musical Expression of Moodstates," *Psychology of Music* 19 (1991): 99–109.

Thaut and de l'Etoile, 1993.

[2]A. L. Bouhuys, G. M. Bloem, and T. G. Groothius, "Induction of Depressed and Elated Mood by Music Influences the Perception of Facial Emotional Expressions in Healthy Subjects," *Journal of Affective Disorders* 33/4 (1995): 215–26.

[3]Pignatiello, 1989.

[4]VanderArk and Ely, 1993.

[5]National Institute of Mental Health, 1996.

[6]Ben Green and Chris Dowrick, "Depression," *Psychiatry in General Practice*, ed. Ben Green (Dordrecht and Boston: Kluwer Academic, 1994).

Terence Real, *I Don't Want to Talk About It* (New York: Scribner, 1997).

Myrna M. Weissman, Martha Livingston Bruce, Phillip J. Leaf, Louis P. Florio, and Charles Holzer III, "Affective Disorders," *Psychiatric Disorders in America: The Epidemiologic Catchment*, Lee N. Robin and Darrel A. Regier, eds. (New York: The Free Press, 1991).

[7] Heller, 1987.

[8] Brown and Mankowski, 1993.

[9]G. Martin, M. Clarke, and C. Pearce, "Adolescent Suicide: Music Preference as an Indication of Vulnerability," *Journal of the American Academy of Child and Adolescent Psychiatry* 32/3 (1993): 530–35.

[10]Adaman and Blaney, 1995.

Bouhuys, Bloem, and Groothius, 1995.

[11]Robazza, Macaluso, and D'Urso, 1994.

[12]Tergwot and van Grinsven, 1991.

[13]Chen, 1992.

Green and Dowrick, 1994.

Hanser and Thompson, 1994.

Jochims, 1992.

[14]Sandra Burak-Maholik, "Psychoeducational Strategies for Depressed Students," *Journal of Emotional and Behavioral Problems* 2/2 (1993): 45–47.

[15]Pignatiello, 1989.

[16]S. R. Lenton and P. R. Martin, "The Contribution of Music vs. Instructions in the Musical Mood Induction Procedure," *Behaviour Research and Therapy* 29/6 (1991): 623–25.

Valerie N. Stratton and Annette H. Zalanowski, "The Effects of Music and Paintings on Mood," *Journal of Music Therapy* 26/1 (1989): 30–41.

Stratton and Zalanowski, 1991.

[17]Michael J. Migliore, "The Hamilton Rating Scale for Depression and

Rhythmic Competency: A Correlational Study," *Journal of Music Therapy* 28/4 (1991): 211–21.

[18]Lord and Garner, 1993.

[19]Thaut and de l'Etoile, 1993.

[20]Robazza, Macaluso, and D'Urso, 1994.

Tergwot and van Grinsven, 1991.

[21]Beth Azar, "Intrusive Thoughts Proven to Undermine Our Health," *The APA Monitor* 10/96.

[22]Sharon Begley, "One Pill Makes You Larger, and One Pill Makes You Small," *Newsweek* 2/7/94: 37–43.

[23]Eifert, Craill, Carey, and O'Connor, 1988.

G. Sutherland, B. Newman, and S. Rachman, "Experimental Investigations of the Relations Between Mood and Intrusive Unwanted Cognitions," *British Journal of Medical Psychology* 55 (1982): 127–38.

[24]Begley, 1994.

Michael W. Miller, "Fat Pharm: Respect for Diet Pills Rises as Studies Shed New Light on Obesity," *Wall Street Journal* 7/20/94: A1+.

Elizabeth Somer, *Food and Mood* (New York: Henry Holt, 1995).

[25]Begley, 1994.

[26]L. F. Lowenstein, "The Treatment of Extreme Shyness in Maladjusted Children by Implosive, Counselling, and Conditioning Approaches," *Acta Psychiatrica Scandinavica* 66/3 (1982): 173–89.

[27]Thaut and de l'Etoile, 1993.

[28]F. J. Prerost, "A Strategy to Enhance Humor Production among Elderly Persons: Assisting in the Management of Stress," *Activities, Adaptation and Aging* 17 (1993): 17–24.

David S. Smith, "An Age-Based Comparison of Humor in Selected Musical Compositions," *Journal of Music Therapy* 31/3 (1994): 206–219.

K.F. Tennant, "Laugh It Off: The Effect of Humor on the Well-Being of the Older Adult," *Journal of Gerontological Nursing* 16/12 (1990): 11–17.

Chapter Six

[1]Harris, Bradley, and Titus, 1992.

P. King, "Heavy Metal Music and Drug Abuse in Adolescents," *Postgraduate Medicine* 83/5 (1988): 295–301.

J. D. Klein, J. D. Brown, K. W. Childers, J. Oliveri, C. Porter, and C. Dykers, "Adolescents' Risky Behavior and Mass Media Use," *Pediatrics* 92/1 (1993): 24–31.

Jack B. Moore, *Skinheads: Shaved for Battle. A Cultural History of American Skinheads* (Bowling Green, OH: Bowling Green University Popular Press, 1993).

D. L. Peterson and K. S. Pfost, "Influence of Rock Videos on Attitudes of Violence Against Women." *Psychological Reports* 64/1 (1989): 319–22.

J. G. Pfaus, L. D. Myronuk, and W. J. Jacobs, "Soundtrack Contents and Depicted Sexual Violence," *Archives of Sexual Behavior* 15/3 (1986): 231–37.

B. L. Plopper and M. E. Ness, "Death as Portrayed to Adolescents through Top 40 Rock and Roll Music," *Adolescence* 28/112 (1993): 793–807.

Victor C. Strasburger and Robert L. Hendren, "Rock Music and Music Videos," *Pediatric Annals* 24/2 (1995): 97–103.

Kevin J. Took and David S. Weiss, "The Relationship between Heavy Metal and Rap Music and Adolescent Turmoil: Real or Artifact?" *Adolescence* 29/115 (1994): 613–21.

Bruce H. Wade, "Explicit Rap Music Lyrics and Attitudes toward Rape: The Perceived Effects on African American College Students' Attitudes," *Challenge: A Journal of Research on African American Men* 4/1 (1993): 51–60.

B. M. Waite, M. Hillbrand, and H. G. Foster, "Reduction of Aggressive Behavior after Removal of Music Television," *Hospital and Community Psychiatry* 43/2 (1992): 173–75.

[2]D. S. Berry and J. W. Pennebaker, "Nonverbal and Verbal Emotional Expression and Health," *Psychotherapy and Psychosomatics* 59/1 (1993): 11–19.

[3]M. Fava, M. Abraham, J. Pava, J. Shuester, and J. Rosenbaum, "Cardiovascular Risk Factors in Depression: The Role of Anxiety and Anger," *Psychosomatics* 37/1 (1996): 31–37.

L. Keltikangas-Järvinen, K. Räikkönen, A. Hautanen, and H. Adlercreutz, "Vital Exhaustion, Anger Expression, and Pituitary and Adrenocortical Hormones: Implications for the Insulin Resistance Syndrome," *Arteriosclerosis, Thrombosis, and Vascular Biology* 16/2 (1996): 275–80.

[4]Erin Burnett, "Anger Undercuts Ethnic-Minority Women's Health," *The APA Monitor* 10/96.

[5]J. G. Beck and A. W. Bozman, "Gender Differences in Sexual Desire: The Effects of Anger and Anxiety," *Archives of Sexual Behavior* 24/6 (1995): 595–612.

[6]Berry and Pennebaker, 1993.

[7]M. M. Müller, H. Rau, S. Brody, T. Elbert, and H. Heinle, "The Rela-

tionship Between Habitual Anger Coping Style and Serum Lipid and Lipoprotein Concentrations," *Biological Psychology* 41/1 (1995): 69–81.

[8]Klein et al., 1993.

[9]Took and Weiss, 1994.

[10]Peterson and Pfost, 1989.

[11]Pfaus, Myronuk, and Jacobs, 1986.

[12]Wade, 1993.

[13]Peterson and Pfost, 1989.

Pfaus, Myronuk, and Jacobs, 1986.

Strasburger, 1995.

Waite, Hillbrand, and Foster, 1992.

[14]Heather Aldridge and Diana B. Carlin, "The Rap on Violence: A Rhetorical Analysis of Rapper KRS-One," *Communication Studies* 44/2 (1993): 102–16.

[15]Altschuler, 1948.

Gatewood, 1921.

Mathews, 1806.

Shatin, 1970.

[16]The discussion of anger in this chapter draws upon American Psychological Association, "Controlling Anger—Before It Controls You," Washington, DC, nd.

[17]Frances F. Cripe, "Rock Music as Therapy for Children with Attention Deficit Disorder: An Exploratory Study," *Journal of Music Therapy* 23/1 (1986): 30–37.

[18]Burnett, 1996.

[19]A. Caraveli-Chaves, "Bridge Betweeen Words: The Greek Woman's Lament as Communicative Event," *Journal of American Folklore* 93 (1980): 129–41.

Steven Feld, *Sound and Sentiment: Birds, Weeping, Poetics, and Song in Kaluli Expression* (Philadelphia: University of Pennsylvania Press, 1982).

Laura Graham, "Three Modes of Shavante Vocal Expression: Wailing, Collective Singing, and Political Oratory," *Native South American Discourse,* Joel Sherzer and Greg Urban, eds. (Berlin: Mouton de Gruyter, 1986).

Margarita Mazo, "Lament Made Visible: A Study of Paramusical Elements in Russian Lament," *Themes and Variations: Writings on Music in Honor of Rulan Chao Pian,* Bell Yung and Joseph S. C. Lam, eds. (Cambridge and Hong Kong: Department of Music, Harvard University and The Institute of Chinese Studies, The Chinese University of Hong Kong, 1994): 164–211.

Elizabeth Tolbert, "Women Cry with Words: Symbolization of Affect in the Karelian Lament," *Yearbook for Traditional Music* 22 (1990): 80–105.

Greg Urban, "Ritual Wailing in Amerindian Brazil," *American Anthropologist* 90 (1988): 385–400.

[20] Jochims, 1992.

[21] Pierre Charles Morin, "Evaluation of Depression Reconsidered: A Qualitative Analysis of Franz Schubert's WinterReise," paper presented at the Second International Conference on Music Perception and Cognition, Los Angeles, CA, 1992.

Chapter Seven

[1] Edward de Bono, *Serious Creativity: Using the Power of Lateral Thinking to Create New Ideas* (New York: Harper Business, 1992).

Tony Buzan, *Use Both Sides of Your Brain* (New York: E. P. Dutton, 1991).

Betty Edwards, *Drawing on the Right Side of the Brain: A Course in Enhancing Creativity and Artistic Confidence* (J. P. Tarcher, 1989).

Michael Michalko, *Thinkertoys: A Handbook of Business Creativity for the 90s* (Berkeley: Ten Speed Press, 1991).

Roger von Oech, *A Whack on the Side of the Head: How You Can Be More Creative* (Menlo Park, CA: Creative Think, 1983).

Robert W. Olson, *The Art of Creative Thinking* (New York: Barnes and Noble, 1980).

Alex Osborn, *Applied Imagination* (New York: Scribner, 1963).

Joyce Wycoff, *Mindmapping: Your Personal Guide to Exploring Creativity and Problem Solving* (New York: Berkley Books, 1991).

[2] E. Paul Torrance and Kathy Goff, "Fostering Creativity in Gifted Students," *ERIC Digest* 484 (1990).

[3] Adaman and Blaney, 1995.

Bill Kaltsounis, "Effect of Sound on Creative Performance," *Psychological Reports* 33/3 (1973): 737–38.

Cathy H. McKinney and Frederick C. Tims, "Differential Effects of Selected Classical Music on the Imagery of High Versus Low Imagers: Two Studies," *Journal of Music Therapy* 22/1 (1995): 22–45.

[4] Torrance and Goff, 1990.

[5] Jourdain, 1997.

[6] Osborn, 1993.

[7] Kaltsounis, 1973.

[8] McKinney and Tims, 1995.

[9]Maurice Sendak, "The Shape of Music," *Caldecott & Co.* (The Noonday Press, 1990): 4.

[10]Buzan, 1991.

Wycoff, 1991.

[11]Betty Edwards, *Drawing on the Artist Within: An Inspirational and Practical Guide to Increasing Your Creative Powers* (New York: Fireside, 1987).

[12]McLaughlin, 1970.

[13]Helen L. Bonny, "Music and Consciousness," *Journal of Music Therapy* 12/3 (1975): 121–35.

[14]Bonny, 1975.

[15]Adaman and Blaney, 1995.

[16]S. Zagona and M. Kelly, "The Resistance of the Closed Mind to a Novel and Complex Audio-Visual Experience," *Journal of Social Psychology* 70 (1966): 123–31.

[17]von Oech, 1983.

[18]de Bono, 1992.

[19]Greer, 1980.

[20]R. M. Moyle, "Sexuality in Samoan Art Forms," *Archives of Sexual Behavior* 4/3 (1975): 227–47.

[21]Zagona and Kelly, 1966.

[22]Beckett, 1990.

[23]Kaltsounis, 1973.

[24]Valerie N. Stratton and Annette H. Zalanowski, "The Effects of Music and Cognition on Mood," *Psychology of Music* 19 (1991): 121–7.

Start Tuning Your
BRAIN
NOW

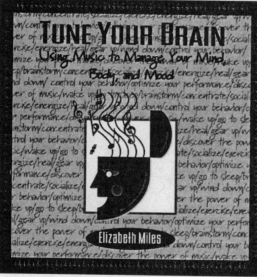

(DG: 457 356-2/4)

Discover
the Power
of Classical
Music.

Take the Mood Journey
Created by Elizabeth Miles and
the World's Leading Classical Label:
Deutsche Grammophon

Available on CD and Cassette at fine record stores everywhere or by calling 1-800-40-MUSIC.

a PolyGram company